Stopping Military Suicides

Stopping Military Suicides

VETERAN VOICES TO HELP PREVENT DEATHS

Kate Hendricks Thomas and Sarah Plummer Taylor

Foreword by Patrick McGuigan

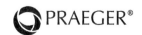

PRAEGER®

An Imprint of ABC-CLIO, LLC
Santa Barbara, California • Denver, Colorado

Library of Congress Cataloging-in-Publication Data

Names: Thomas, Kate Hendricks, author. | Taylor, Sarah Plummer, author.
Title: Stopping military suicides : veteran voices to help prevent deaths /
  Sarah Plummer Taylor and Kate Hendricks Thomas ; foreword by Patrick
  McGuigan.
Description: Santa Barbara : Praeger, an imprint of ABC-CLIO, 2021. | Includes bibliographical
  references and index.
Identifiers: LCCN 2020027355 (print) | LCCN 2020027356 (ebook) | ISBN
  9781440875076 (hardcover) | ISBN 9781440875083 (ebook)
Subjects: LCSH: Veterans—Suicidal behavior—United States. |
  Veterans—Mental health services—United States. | Suicide—United
  States—Prevention. | Post-traumatic stress
  disorder—Patients—Treatment.
Classification: LCC HV6545.7 .T46 2021 (print) | LCC HV6545.7 (ebook) |
  DDC 362.28/7086970973—dc23
LC record available at https://lccn.loc.gov/2020027355
LC ebook record available at https://lccn.loc.gov/2020027356

ISBN: 978-1-4408-7507-6 (print)
      978-1-4408-7508-3 (ebook)

25 24 23 22 21   1 2 3 4 5

This book is also available as an eBook.

Praeger
An Imprint of ABC-CLIO, LLC

ABC-CLIO, LLC
147 Castilian Drive
Santa Barbara, California 93117
www.abc-clio.com

This book is printed on acid-free paper ∞

Manufactured in the United States of America

To my beloved family and next-door neighbors, Lynn and Matt.
Thank you for being there for us the way you always have and
for being such a gift to Matthew.
Kate Hendricks Thomas

To my husband, Pete. You are my rock.
To my daughters, Lila and Brennan. Thank you for
choosing me as your mother.
Sarah Plummer Taylor

Contents

Trigger Warning

The topics covered in this book may be disturbing to some readers. Therefore, we want to share in advance that there will be discussions of suicide, mental health issues, and military sexual trauma in this book. Strong reactions are normal, and we understand that choosing what to read and what to skip is personal. Please practice self-care as you decide whether or not to read the science and stories in the coming pages. This book is not intended as medical advice, diagnosis, or treatment. As always, if you feel a need for resources, call the National Suicide Prevention hotline at 1(800)-273-8255. Veterans can access mental health resources at that phone number and identify as military-affiliated/veteran by pressing 1.

Foreword: Community-Focused Solutions for Veteran Suicide Prevention

Patrick McGuigan

One cannot begin to solve a problem until it is understood; in order to understand it, you need to first identify and admit that you have a problem. This book identifies and explores the public health problem of veteran suicide, offering solutions through a community approach that cements the individual veteran at the center. With more than seven thousand veterans and servicemembers taking their lives every year for almost a decade, one can make a strong argument that we not only have a problem but also a crisis. Over the past ten years, federal funding increased by $6 billion and mental health care became more accessible, especially at the point of crisis in an attempt to reduce and prevent veteran suicide. This approach, although meaningful, achieved no effect in reducing and preventing veterans from taking their lives.

This book is about how to best identify the problem and begin to address it. A community-first approach, where everything begins, operates, and excels in and through the community, sets the foundation to finally address the problem before individual crisis. A community solution that enhances outreach through social and peer engagement, presented in a wrap-around resource manner, enables an upstream prevention model by offering a smooth transition back to civilian life. For the past ten years, programs and organizations viewed themselves as the sun, expecting the veteran to orbit around them. A true community approach, as described in this book, will place the veteran as the sun within the community and have organizations and resources orbit around them. It also considers the role the active duty component can play in getting veterans prepared for transition by strengthening individual levels of resilience prior to service separation.

My perspective was shaped and developed over the past eighteen months while traveling the country meeting with people and organizations, living and working in their communities. Consistently engaging with organizations helping veterans at the grassroots, tactical level provided me with a grounded perspective. In a unique way, learning about community interventions to prevent veteran suicide reminded me of my almost thirty months of conducting counterinsurgency (COIN) operations during the surges in Iraq and Afghanistan. My days were filled with meetings with village leaders and elders trying to establish and maintain security for the locals. There, I would walk the villages to capture the atmospherics and underlying issues that caused insecurity. Here, I was in the community trying to gain atmospherics and an understanding for what was triggering so many veterans to take their lives. What both of those experiences had in common was the realization that you truly cannot understand the issue and begin to address it until you live in and become part of the community. In addition to efforts within the DOD and Department of Veterans Affairs (VA), the resources of the local community must be part of any meaningful solution in the future.

As I parachuted into public service after over a decade of active duty military service, I approached the problem set from a perspective not as a doctor, mental health professional, scientist, or researcher, but rather from a leadership perspective. Through my public-service related travels, I consistently thought about how to get leadership from the private and public sectors at the national, state, and local levels more engaged on the issue. The takeaway from this observation is engaged leadership must exist, operate, and thrive in the community. The best community models had strong synergy of leadership in the community between private and public organizations. It is through these strong partnerships that enable communities to set a foundation allowing for a veteran's smooth transition into civilian life. This transition is the critical first step to prevent suicide.

A smooth transition into the community is vital for a veteran and their family to start the new chapter in life on a positive trajectory. A transition supported by a community where its existing veterans and organizations provide means and ways to connect and join their tribe is an upstream way of preventing suicide. Strong, resilient communities provide an organized and synchronized approach to navigating and finding resources within the community to support the transition of a veteran. However, just because you have resources available does not mean they are effective in supporting the veteran's transition. The resources need to be presented and offered in an organized manner, precisely applied at the appropriate time and in the right mechanism under accountable means in order to achieve the effect for which they are purposed.

With more veterans currently dying due to suicide each year than servicemembers deployed in support of the global war on terror, one can argue that transition is more dangerous than being deployed today. How can this be possible? Servicemembers spend a year or longer training with the same team in preparing to be deployed. Everyone knows their role and their responsibility; muscle memory is created on how to react to every possible situation. This allows the team to become a tribe and ensures everyone within the tribe knows exactly their role and responsibility; it creates a sense of self-worth and self-identity for every individual. There is no lengthy training provided by the military for transition, and in fairness, that is not the military's job. It is up to the individual to develop a transition plan for post military life. Every veteran knows that no plan ever survives first contact, and this includes the best transition plan. The problem is, when the transition plan comes under attack, unlike the muscle memory established to know how to react to contact, there is no muscle memory for reacting to contact as a civilian. This often triggers internal reflection of self-worth.

A strong community can enhance and create a strong sense of belonging, leading to a newly discovered and fortified sense of self-worth. This self-worth drives self-purpose and belief that you do have a place and purpose in a tribe, a new tribe, a community tribe. Veterans offer an experience and perspective that 99 percent of their peers and fellow citizens do not. Strong communities know how to leverage and promote that experience to better the community and its people. Communities that enable veterans to find their new self-worth and value will promote the renewed sense of self-purpose and work to prevent veterans and others in the community from ever reaching a point of crisis.

The experience of working in a military professional organization that instills goal-orientated values in oneself cements a belief that the cause is greater than oneself; it is an unparalleled and powerful asset not only to a community but also to the society. The more we can leverage that mentality and those experiences, helping veterans understand the critical role they play in society, the stronger our community becomes. The second-order effect of this is the potential to reduce and prevent suicide. Communities can eliminate stigmas and positively encourage veterans through the nonclinical decision-making experience that often leads to getting mental health care. The community is the first line of defense to suicide; the better the understanding to leverage and utilize community to address the issue of suicide, the better the chance we have to understand the problem and fix it.

1

Author's Note: The Pistol or the Yoga Mat

Sarah Plummer Taylor

I was 26 years old in January of 2007 when I found myself sitting alone, in my can—my room—in Iraq. I had a choice to make, one of the most important choices of my life.

During my time in service, I was a very typical Marine in many ways. I worked hard, trained hard, played hard. I was an Intelligence Officer who served about seven years of active duty, including two deployments to Iraq, and when I left the military, I did some volunteer work in the Middle East and Europe. Upon my return to the States, I worked for an intelligence agency in Washington, D.C., for a while and then spent most of the last eight plus years running a business that supports executive teams, entrepreneurs, and veterans who want to improve the quality of their lives and leadership. Under this business's scope, I also work as a pediatric sleep consultant and family wellness counselor.

Now, in 2020, I call myself a "veteran," and I am so fortunate to be the mother of an adorable human named Lila, who is expecting a sister soon, as well as a dog mom to my fur babies. I'm a wife, a daughter, a sister, friend, lifelong student, outdoor lover, and a small business owner.

That could sum it up. I could paint this picture of an easy transition from leadership in the military to leadership principles that I teach and apply in my work and business now, and you'd be none the wiser to know that, actually, at several points in my life I've almost been on the other side of things. Because the truth is, both my entry into *and* out of the military was anything but smooth. That is the case for many of us veterans; I am not special in that regard.

We veterans are a unique, talented, and resilient group of people who the world needs to keep getting to know better! We can be such assets to our communities, our families, and each other. We are not a homogenous group, so talking about us *and* resilience-building is a multilayered discussion, and the solutions to some of our most pressing challenges involve a complex combination of systemic change and civic support plus individual resilience practices. And I know all about the pressure and temptation to be too busy taking care of others to take care of myself. But when we do that, we rob our families, our workplace, our communities, and our friends from experiencing our most creative, confident, and compassionate selves, and ultimately, that stifles our resilience-building and can prevent us from making our highest contribution to the world.

Now the funny thing is, I was actually in Air Force training my first two years in college, but I secretly wished to be a Marine. The summer between my second and third years in college, that desire was no longer so secret when I confirmed my choice to switch branches.

However, this intent to switch set off a string of cautionary lectures from not only the Air Force leadership at my school but also through letters and phone calls from my recently retired Air Force father, who said he would never approve of this decision and that I was ruining my life. This is part of one of his letters to me, one week before 9/11. He said:

> I will never say I approve of your decision to join the Marines. And thank God, you will never have to fight in a war, but there is death and destruction you'll have to deal with. . . . Please don't do this.

Many of the things my father warned me of happened, as well as others of which he didn't dare speak but knew to be very possible. My mother, too, made many comments strongly disapproving of my choice to be in the military at all. For many women and men, choosing the military—or a specific branch over another—is a hugely countercultural choice either within our immediate families and or within our larger communities of identity. It's not always a celebrated traditional path for everyone.

But in my gut, in my heart, I knew the Marines was where I was supposed to be, and so ultimately, it was an authentic choice—as hard as it was to make, as vulnerable as I had to be to make it—it was a choice I could live with, even when those terrible things that my father was afraid of happened.

We've all been in a situation when we thought we might disappoint someone we love because of the choices we make about our particular path. Yet, to continue to live in a way that is out of alignment with who we are at our very core, to live *inauthentically*, can destroy us.

Sometimes those feared disappointments are around big things like career, education, or family, and sometimes they're seemingly small but equally impactful day-to-day choices about how we care for ourselves *or not*. If you're living life based on other people's expectations, or running yourself ragged in the name of success, or *even in the name of serving others*, you're not doing anyone any favors. You're likely too tired to even know who your authentic self really is or what your intuition is telling you.

I know because I did that, and I've seen so many of my military friends do it. I shut down my intuitive wisdom after years of striving to blend in with the men around me, sacrificing my individual identity for the greater good of the unit like we all often did, and living the kind of extreme reality that military culture tends to reward.

And because I thought resilience meant running more, lifting more, doing more, working more, and pushing myself beyond my own limits and to just keep going through all of that, that's what I did. I thought that was resilience: just keep going.

Somewhere along the way though, after sucking it up for years, I lost the will to keep fighting.

My body was shutting down.

My heart was breaking.

And one morning, during my second deployment to Iraq, as I lay on my cot, alone, in my room, my eyes opened.

It would be a lie to say I awoke in bed in these morning moments because I went days at a time without actually sleeping. I had racing thoughts about experiences during that deployment. I had nightmares. I was still utterly heartbroken about my marriage that had painfully ended a few years before. And the physical pain I was in from a variety of musculoskeletal and head injuries, as well as stress injuries, kept me in a constant state of wincing. I was in my 20s, looked like I was in my 30s or 40s, and felt like I was in my 80s.

The first thing I saw was my pistol. Just a simple, black, standard Marine Corps issue M9 pistol. It was hanging on my bedpost, in the brown leather holster that my ex-boyfriend had given me. (Because those are the kind of gifts you give a loved one when you're in the Marines.)

And I also saw my $20 yoga mat, beige, almost the same color of the sand I was always surrounded by, rolled up, at the foot of my bed between it and my wall locker.

That room was big enough for a wall locker, a single bed, and a yoga mat to be rolled out on the floor next to it.

I blinked.

It was excruciating to exist.

And I thought to myself, "It would just be easier if I wasn't here."

And I had a choice: the pistol or the yoga mat.

It was life or death.

We *all* have these moments when we have to make *big choices*. When we find ourselves in battle zones feeling completely alone. If and when we feel that we are alone, or that we don't know who we are, or that we have no purpose, we end up *choosing death* literally or symbolically. We give up. Or we check out. And loneliness kills.

Instead of holding our breath, holding back, holding it all in, or waiting, what if we got on our "yoga mat" and started to breathe? What if our inhales and exhales weren't things we took for granted but those that we used to direct our very essence, our focus, our purpose, our intuition, our intention, attention, and connection?

Inhale. Exhale.

I had an epiphany then that has stuck with me since: my breath was mine; it was the one thing no one could touch. At a time when I felt like every single aspect of my life had someone else's hands on it, they couldn't touch my breath.

The reality is everyone has had a difficult choice to make. Mine was life or death. Many of yours would have been life or death.

We have the pistol choice we can make or the yoga mat choice we can make.

Like staying on the couch for another hour of TV or getting up to go outside for a little walk or a jog. The pistol or the yoga mat?

Like having the same argument with our partner over and over again or choosing to give counseling a try. The pistol or the yoga mat?

Like housing a pint of ice cream at midnight, straight from the carton, standing there with the freezer door open, when you are exhausted and not thinking straight versus doing your best to eat a healthy dinner and then actually going to bed when you're tired. The pistol or the yoga mat?

We always have a choice.

Resilience gives us choice.

So, how do we do it now? How do we narrow things down from all the choices we have?

The good news is that the evidence base is so rich now that it shows us that resilience—across populations—is built upon three empirically validated pillars: social support, self-care, and spiritual practices. When all three are combined, their power is magnified.

The resilience-building that helps military personnel and veterans helps us all be better parents, partners, employees, bosses, or friends.

So throughout this book, we will share the evidence-based components to resilience-building that benefit *all* of us. My hope is that through hearing these concepts, you can personalize and specify resilience-building into your life because it equips us all to lead, love, and live to our fullest potential without burning out.

2

Author's Note: A Culture of Silence

Kate Hendricks Thomas

My story started the way many do, with sparkly attraction that morphed into friendship and then into love. It was the sort of love that changed the way one saw the world. Unfortunately, my story also ended the way too many do, with holes in the walls, broken doors, and police knocking at the front door.

I met Kyle by accident—I hadn't even planned to go out to dinner with my friends that evening. I walked up to the table with hair casually tossed into a ponytail and zero expectations. He smiled at me, and he had a smile that seemed to light up the room. I remember that being my first impression—a wide grin and lots of very white teeth. There was a knowing in our eye contact, and it seemed like the decision to become inseparable was made for us both in that instant. Kyle made me laugh at every turn. He was charming and outgoing—the life of every party.

We were both Marine officers, which meant he understood my work world. I can't tell you how ridiculous it was to try to date a civilian guy as a Marine; I got so many crazy comments, odd looks, or would-be boyfriends who couldn't understand why I was *still* at the office. My job demanded long hours at least six days per week. I often slept in the field or had over-night duty, and it was a relief to spend time with a man who understood a schedule like that.

We worked hard and played even harder, which was all perfectly normal in the Marine Corps. Free time was a rare commodity, making us feel like every night out should be as epic as possible. We were sensation seekers who were always up for a challenge or adventure. To us, epic nights out often meant heavy drinking and keeping late hours at bars.

Kyle and I got serious quickly. A lot of us on active duty did that. Someone was always being deployed, and those outside circumstances often forced big questions and placed premature pressures on military relationships. Soon after we started dating, Kyle was packing bags to head overseas again, and we had to make quick decisions about what we were to one another. Moving in together, getting married, and spending as much time together as the Marine Corps allowed wove the tapestry of our early relationship, and we were at once both wild and wildly happy.

It is hard to explain what my tie to Kyle felt like. He was the first person I had shared almost everything with, and he was never judgmental. The guardedness that characterized my professional life of course seeped into my personal life, and I had always shown boyfriends incomplete versions of myself. For someone unaccustomed to sharing, doing so felt cathartic and bred feelings of closeness that allowed me to ignore certain things.

First came the red flags that I ignored because I had all the same problems. Kyle drank in binge fashion, early and often. He was reckless and took risks at any opportunity, always up for some untried, new experience. Most of the time I was right there with him. If you only had one day off or were counting down the days until your next overseas rotation, it didn't seem unreasonable to drink all day long or find something crazy to do in order to maximize your limited playtime.

Then there were the flags that I somehow chose to ignore and excuse because I was blindly smitten. Kyle would mix prescription pain medication with alcohol or go out late and head to work without sleeping at all. One night he was gone until 4.00 a.m., and he couldn't explain where he had been. He had dark periods of time when he would disappear into himself, crawling into bed for days and taking NyQuil to stay asleep.

It still seems embarrassing to admit out loud that I didn't see the downhill slide. I was at once too busy and too proud. At the time, I didn't see Kyle's behaviors as symptomatic of anything more than boredom or a bad attitude, and I railed against each one with righteous anger. It became a cycle of fights, promises, and forgiveness, which was always on repeat.

I also stayed very good at keeping up appearances. When one of his angry outbursts left a foot-sized hole in our wall, I moved furniture and arranged pictures to cover the damage. When family and friends came to visit, I had clever explanations for why the doors in our house were off the hinges. Loud yelling became shoves into walls or furniture.

Our fashionable apartment and put-together life started coming apart, and my self-denial got harder to keep up. One sunny afternoon, he dragged me across the living room floor by my hair and threw me out the front door. I remember being glad that our industrial-style concrete floors were smooth and polished—at least I slid easily. I can't even recall why he was angry. The neighbors who called the police never asked me any questions, and I never offered them anything but averted eyes. I couldn't tell anyone about it, even as forgiving and forgetting each incident was getting harder and harder to do. I was all alone at this point by choice. I was too invested in seeming smart at all times, and I knew smart women weren't supposed to have problems like these in their relationships.

The influence of culture on my behavior during that period of time and on behavior in general cannot be understated. It never entered my mind that Kyle had a problem with depression or stress injury and that all of his self-medication had a source. It never entered my mind to go ask someone for help with an abusive relationship that kept escalating.

Never.

I'm a freaking Amazon. A Marine. These things don't happen in my world.

I had a choice in my situation, but as a Marine, my culture was one of independence and infallibility. Only the weak had problems, and my husband and I couldn't be weak.

As things got worse in our home, I was truly not equipped to be a real source of help to Kyle. I was as invested in presenting an image of strong silence as he was, trained and driven to disregard symptoms that were staring me right in the face. Warrior subculture tends to promote the belief that acknowledging emotional pain is synonymous with weakness and, specifically, that asking for help for emotional distress or problems is unacceptable.

I've got this.

The result of such a firmly entrenched value system is feeling a whole lot of shame associated with emotional struggle, patient identity, and mental health conditions. They are simply not options. This doesn't just mean that servicemembers deny needing help; it means that we avoid recognizing symptoms as such in ourselves or in those we are close to. If forced to address displayed symptoms, we will take denial to new heights and even actively dodge treatment when prescribed.

I was a leader who had directed Marines working for me to Family Services or Combat Stress many times. But using them myself? Not an option.

Both card-carrying warrior culture members who adhered rigidly to all its norms and values, Kyle and I became a dysfunctional duo in the last year we were together. We both ignored symptoms and put Band-Aids on wounds that were both figurative and literal.

Kyle's personality was unpredictable. He would go from being really energetic to very withdrawn or even angry and violent without warning. One long weekend, he canceled our plans to see friends. He went to bed for four days and wouldn't speak or even get up to eat. I stayed nearby, confused and worried, hoping to cajole him into a happier mood. I didn't call anyone.

I'm not a psychiatrist, but to this day, I cannot believe that I didn't recognize his symptoms. I knew he had the mood swings and sleeplessness that often come along with a depression diagnosis, but I never pushed counseling—that was something those other weak people needed. I never associated him with mental illness or considered it a possibility. I never asked myself if my own angry mental state or feelings of alienation were healthy.

Our days were very, very dark toward the end. They were a haze of alcohol and bad choices, walking on eggshells, crying, and making shameful compromises.

This isn't me.

This can't be who I am.

Is this the future I choose?

My best friend was disappearing into a sad place right in front of my eyes, and I didn't know how to see that reality, much less help him. Alcoholic, addict, depressed, unstable—these were all labels I couldn't bring myself to apply to him. I was both ill-equipped and too close to help. No matter how much I read about codependent behavior or how often I hear differently, it still feels like a failure, a label that I will always carry.

I was afraid in my own home, but I would never have labeled myself a victim of anything. I had no idea yet that I needed help and wouldn't have known how to accept it if someone had offered.

It wasn't until one of Kyle's particularly scary benders left me alone in our apartment, searching for places to hide our ammunition, when I realized something had to change. He was mixing alcohol with Valium at the time, and I could barely understand his speech. He had become paranoid, obsessively checking my whereabouts, phone records, and e-mail inbox.

I had no idea where he had gone that night, but I knew he always came back drunk. I searched for places to hide away rounds so that even if he went for one of our weapons when he came home, he wouldn't have anything with which to fire them. I knew he needed help, and a tiny doubt began to creep into my mind about whether I was ever going to be able to get him to seek it before something bad happened to me. It was the first time I considered leaving, knowing I might be leaving him drowning.

Servicemembers are conditioned to avoid recognizing symptoms that could indicate depression or post-traumatic stress. This makes perfect sense when considering the unique and treatment-recalcitrant military culture in which this phenomenon occurs. Mental health conditions are viewed as moral failures and civilian treatment providers as benevolent but untrusted outsiders. We don't want to see depression or post-traumatic stress symptoms in ourselves, in those we love, and we certainly don't wish to seek professional help.

The results of our belief system show up in our suicide statistics. Before the wars in Iraq and Afghanistan, the incidence of suicide in active duty U.S. servicemembers was consistently 25 percent lower than in the civilian population. Currently, military and veteran suicide rates exceed those found in the general population.

Providers work tirelessly to dream up new ways to treat depression and stress injury, but they can only ever provide a partial solution. The answer can't come solely in treatment form.

Too many of us won't recognize the need for professional help, seek it out, or stick with treatment if forced to go. It becomes easier to wall ourselves off from the world than to share vulnerabilities or shameful imperfections.

Without ever making any of these admissions, I filed divorce papers and packed the car. I called Kyle's sister and left her a message that asked her to look out for him without giving away any in-depth information. I was still being loyal, in my own mind. I left everything material I owned at our former home with him and drove off, a completely broken version of myself.

The years to come would be tough ones, but I made choices to dig myself out from under the grief and depression. Professional counseling was part of the equation, but what really made the biggest difference was stumbling across the components of resiliency. I learned through experience and academic study that specific traits make a person more bulletproof, and I wanted some of that, whatever I had to do. I couldn't change the influences that made my transition from military service and my marriage so hard, but I saw an opportunity to do things differently in the future. For me, that was the beginning of better.

What if I had known how to build my own resilience long before I needed it? Keep reading because that knowledge might make a difference for you and yours', too.

SECTION 1

Introduction to the Battlespace

3

Overview of the Issues

Despite the vast news coverage of the wars in Iraq and Afghanistan since 2001, one figure has remained mysterious: the number of suicides among U.S. servicemen and women compared with combat casualties. Right now, we are losing more military personnel to suicide than to combat. Veteran suicides have become a public health crisis, and impact all service eras, races, sexualities, and genders. For example, women veterans are 250 percent more likely than civilian women to die by suicide.

Those figures are mysterious because even as we throw money and resources at clinical mental health treatment and blame rising rates on multiple deployments, the answers are elusive. The narrative of the "broken veteran" struggling with combat stress just doesn't ring quite true to those of us who have served over the last decade, and the issue is more complicated than simple statistics can show.

We became Marines to serve, and we have loved being part of the Corps. As with anything ever loved intensely, the military changed and shaped us. To the casual observer looking in, the world seems brutal and intense. That casual observer isn't entirely wrong—the military is some of those things. Shared hardship and challenge are vital parts of the refining and rebuilding process that changes a civilian into a warrior.

That process of obstacles, mastery experience, and shared suffering offers growth and transformation, but coming back to civilian life afterward can be incredibly hard. Standards are different. Camaraderie is different. Culture is absolutely different. We witnessed firsthand the toll that leaving the service took on many of us. Stressful work environments, high rates of divorce and domestic violence, family separation, and repeated combat deployments all contributed, but the biggest reason for the reintegration problems many of us faced was cultural. We subscribe to unbalanced notions of what it means to be a warrior and uphold silent suffering as virtue. Mistakes are shameful; pain is weakness. Saying something is hard or stressful just isn't done.

As veterans, parents, and writers, we don't want to contribute to the silence that surrounds these issues anymore. Too many aspects of warrior culture are destructive lies we tell ourselves.

Constant invulnerability is an illusion, and cultural mandates to be "together" in every way become dangerously prescriptive. We lose our authenticity in this way; we don't know how to reach out to each other when stresses start to overwhelm. Too many of us who are used to appearing strong would, indeed, rather consider suicide than admit to being human, fallible, or broken.

Our own public stories were of crisp uniforms, physical fitness metrics, and successes. We always looked good on paper. The private stories involved a great deal more nuance.

As Marine Officers, we were not supposed to make mistakes, feel depressed, or need help. But we did. Tough places and situations became tougher because we didn't know that people might be okay with an imperfect version of us.

When serving in the military, we are trained to lead with confidence. Presenting a certain and effective facade requires some incredibly useful skills. We make decisions quickly and responsively, but these very same skills become incredibly destructive when we never learn how to turn them off. This description fits most servicemembers. We tend to be a driven, almost comically dysfunctional lot.

What is so useful about sharing our experiences with one another is that we offer each other the opportunity to say that kindest of phrases— "me too." Our stories aren't heroic or rare, and they are only worth sharing in these pages because our lack of resilience when it mattered is so common.

In writing this, we place trust in fellow veterans and in a larger community of people who want to make things better for transitioning servicemembers. This conversation is for you. From clinicians to community volunteers, there is a tribe of supportive people out there who want to help. This conversation is also for you.

When we talk about suicide rates and how we can make things better, we typically talk about designing programs, whether we're operating in the Department of Veterans Affairs (VA) or in the nimble nonprofit sector of

Veteran Service Organizations. Some programs are on point and some miss the mark. Too many don't get evaluated at all, or we count the "number of veterans served" as a successful outcome metric that warrants funding. Spoiler, friends—that number doesn't mean true impact or efficacy.

There are good reasons health professionals advocate for peer-led interventions grounded in resiliency theory. Those reasons are partially based on evaluation metrics and research, but they are also based on the embodied knowledge of veterans who have made the rocky transition and come out on the other side.

The determined avoidance of care-seeking we lived through is disturbingly normal in the military community that we once called home. For us, learning to do better meant stumbling by accident into the three key components required to build human resilience. The answer had always been there; we just hadn't known it when we needed to.

We are killing ourselves alone in apartments, and no one is seeing any symptoms—we are that good at hiding out. It really isn't that services aren't available to veterans and military personnel when things become difficult—we just won't use them. Existing gaps in mental health service provision are created largely by stigma against seeking care.

No matter what magic we do in the clinical realm, focusing on treatment requires a disempowerment narrative that is perceived as being incompatible with the cultural values of military veterans. We cannot overcome such norms by asking warriors to become patients and pop pills, no matter how dedicated, innovative, and gifted the clinician is. While treatment is certainly part of the solution, it is not culturally acceptable for it to be the entire answer.

We know this to be true on both an academic and a personal level—it is embodied knowledge—and believe we need to alter the dialogue about resilience.[1] We must flip the current paradigm and turn words that currently connote weakness (such as authenticity, self-care practices, and social cohesion) into training mandates and metrics of performance.

There is tremendous work to be done.

Mental fitness can be trained and cultivated in each of us. What if upon joining the Marines we had been offered training designed to increase self-awareness and promote resilience? If we had learned to frame self-care as intelligent preparation rather than indulgence, could handling the requisite stresses of returning from a war zone or leaving active duty service been easier?

Post-traumatic stress and depression must be reframed as normal, recoverable conditions rather than diagnoses to ridicule.[2] Regular training and assessment for military personnel can include a mental fitness emphasis, becoming a metric to which all are trained and tested. The research is clear: We need to alter our dialogue about mental health for veterans and focus on resilience as something that can be learned and grown before combat and transition are experienced.

This work is deeply personal to us, and not merely because of our own experiences. We believe passionately in the use of health programming that emphasizes agency and active engagement for veterans to stem the tide of service suicides. We can do this— resilience can be taught. Social support cultivation, self-care modalities, and spiritual practices are the components upon which we must rely, and we must extend a hand to one another rather than overlook existing problems. As veterans, we have to contribute to the solution and cannot look only outside our own community for an answer. A bureaucracy isn't going to ride in and fix everything.

Our generation has served its watch, but we hope we still have something to offer to those who stand guard after us.

NOTES

1. We borrow here from theorist Sandra Harding's writings on embodied knowledge. It is "a way of experiencing a relationship to history, to divinity, to ancestry from within movements of one's own body, from within the deepest memories of one's own cells." Harding, S. (2009). Standpoint theories: Productively controversial. *Hypatia, 24*(4), 192–200.

2. Post-traumatic growth is a phrase with specific meaning. People can grow in radical, positive ways from struggling through hard times. Scholars systematically studying this process and these mechanisms for growth are working on theoretical models that may someday be useful to design programs for trauma sufferers that emphasize strength through adversity. Tedeschi, R. G., & Calhoun, L. G. (2004). Posttraumatic growth: Conceptual foundations and empirical evidence. *Psychological inquiry, 15*(1), 1–18.

4

The Power of Choice

This book is about more than suicide prevention. It is about resilience and post-traumatic growth, moving beyond trauma, and creating a life we love.

What if we lived in a world where people trusted themselves and others, felt connected, and gave themselves grace and patience during difficult transitions? What if, at their core, people knew they had a choice? What if our *veterans* know they have a choice?

We've all heard the statistic: about twenty veterans a day are dying from suicide. It is a crisis; it is heartbreaking, and we have to talk about it regardless of our comfort with the topic. We believe that the stuff that potentially saves veterans from dying by suicide is the same stuff that can help us live optimally. The practices that create resilience offer protective effects and make us a more compassionate parent, a more forgiving and loving partner, a more effective executive, and a more content human being.

Mindful, intentional choice to practice mental fitness as a discipline is the act that transforms the energy of any situation and *keeps* us on a path of resilience, as bumpy as that path may be.

Mindful choice requires awareness, awareness of things that are sometimes very painful, but it's only on the other side of awareness that healing takes place.

We hear a lot about post-traumatic *stress*, but let's think about post-traumatic *growth* and the places where we *do* heal. One of the ways people can heal from trauma is through the vehicle of choice, by cultivating a sense of agency. Growth is possible by choosing to change our relationship with trauma or stress by choosing to move through trauma mindfully, versus avoiding it, burying it, or checking out of life, or remaining stuck in our trauma, repeating the story to ourselves over and over again.

In this book, we do want to talk about choices. This may be a hot button topic in the context in which we will address it because some may say that we cannot choose our life or choose what happens to us after something terrible occurs. *Choice is complex.* There are people who live in marginalized and oppressed segments of our society who have little choice in daily matters that may seem trivial to others. Moreover, there is a lot of human behavior that looks like choice, but in reality, it is the coalescence of a variety of forces acting upon that individual—like genetic factors, environment, race, economics, and otherwise—to lead that person to make choices that may be the best thing they can do in that moment. Some research shows, for instance, some people face barriers due to mental illnesses or other powerful factors that render them incapable of certain choices. Furthermore, especially in the context of trauma, there is much guilt, shame, and self-blame involved in situations in which the victim feels they didn't make the "right" choice in a situation in which they didn't really even have one.

We do not wish to oversimplify a topic as serious as suicide prevention. However, agency and choice can both promote health and well-being. Therefore, our intent with what follows on these pages is not to judge or to compound feelings of guilt. Rather, it is to say this: *in the situations in which the power to choose is available, this book is designed to help.* The fact of the matter is, we are all acting in the best capacity that we can, and the choice may or may not always be available. This book is geared toward empowering us to choose within the moments, within the scope of what's possible, the things that are within our realm of control or our power to change or to choose. Those small choices can create changes. Those changes can create health or increase resilience.

This book's purpose is not to discuss macro-level issues, even though we well understand that they are very important. We believe systemic solutions are possible to those larger challenges, but we feel called to speak to the individual, for whom we *do* believe choice is possible in many moments. We assume that if you've picked this book up, then you are one of those people who has the ability to choose, who has power, and who has responsibility in at least some, if not many, situations. And we believe every one of us has a choice not only every day but also with every single breath.

So, we would like to share a few stories with you about choice. The first story is one that sort of started it all for Sarah, and it is about choice governed by intuition.

It was the summer of 2001. Sarah was in Texas, at Lackland AFB, running up the barracks stairwell with a huge duffel bag on her back, when her left hamstring snapped. A moment in time that she'd been training for, for years (initial officer training), suddenly stood still. Before knowing the exact details of the culprit causing the pain, she knew something had majorly shifted.

Sarah pulled her hamstring on the first day of Air Force Reserve Officer Training Corps (ROTC) field training and then spent five days limping around and muscling through all the events, popping 800 mg Motrins like they were Pez, and going through the motions. The pain never subsided though, and she found herself at a crossroads: whether or not to stay at field training and finish with an injury, which she would've been allowed to do, or ask to return the following year when she was fully healthy.

So less than a week into field training, when the pain became too much to bear, Sarah had to concede that she'd be going home.

She was devastated because when Sarah hurt her leg at Air Force Field Training, it was a shock to her main existence and source of identity in life, which was to succeed at her military training. She felt like she was letting everyone down. But once Sarah got home and had time to process what had happened, she realized, "I can see this obstacle as either something that is going to stop me *or* I can see it as an opportunity or a source of wisdom." Because honestly, the injury was actually a wake-up call. It made Sarah pause, reassess, and reflect. She didn't want to be a victim to her injured leg. So, she saw it as an opening because deep down, intuitively, she knew the Air Force was not for her.

Sarah considers this her earliest, most memorable experience with the "mind-body connection"—not that she would have framed it that way at the time because that would have been too "hippy dippy" from her perspective. Her body was trying to get her attention in a way that her mind couldn't reach her because she'd out-reasoned herself into staying in the Air Force. Her hamstring snap was a wake-up call, one she believed she received both from her sense of a divine power and from her internal self, saying, *"This is not where you're supposed to be."*

A few weeks later, Sarah returned to college and met with both the Marine Corps commanding officer and the Air Force commanding officer of the respective ROTC units and declared her intent to switch services.

It was not an easy thing to do, emotionally or logistically, but it was *possible* because Sarah hadn't completed Air Force Field Training; there was a loophole in the contract that allowed her to switch her commitments. However, this intent to switch set off a string of cautionary lectures from her Air Force leadership as well as letters and phone calls from her parents, including messages from her father saying he would never approve of this decision and that Sarah was ruining her life. This is part of one of his letters to Sarah, his then 20-year-old daughter, one week before 9/11.

The USMC is about ground attack. You will never lead troops in a ground attack (thank God) and that will limit you whether you believe it or not. I've been around all the services. I take the Air Force hands down, and I want only the best for you. I will never say I agree with you becoming a Marine. I *know* the Air Force is a better, more rewarding life. You can believe all you want that you can make it in the macho world of the Marines, that you can make them accept you . . . You will never be a man, you will never be as mean, nasty, tough, strong, etc. The Marines are built on that concept for a reason. It does not matter what they say to be politically correct. They have to believe they are meaner, nastier, and tougher than the enemy bastard whose throat they have to slit on a dark night. We need people like that. Maybe you can do that, maybe you want to do that, but no high-school dropout, weighing 210 pounds with an IQ of 90 is ever going to believe that. I'm sorry if this sounds cruel or perhaps wrong to you, but I know it is true. Should you have the right to prove yourself? Yes. Will you? I doubt it. PFTs are not Iwo Jima's beach where you have a 60lb pack on your back, the water is chest high, the surf is pounding in your face, bullets are whistling around your head, mortars are blowing your unit into hamburger, and you have to turn and say "follow me." Hopefully, you will never have to fight a war, but you are joining (either AF or USMC) to do that if called upon. It's about believing you are right so much that you are willing to do whatever is necessary to win. To kill someone else face-to-face or with a bomb. Decide you can do it. Decide you convince others to do it. About flying. I know from firsthand experience that just wanting to be a pilot isn't enough. I was smart, I was tough, I had more desire than most, but I didn't have enough of whatever to make it. I wasn't a bad person or a failure because of it, but I had to find a different job. So don't ignore this. I'm not trying to jinx you, but you are not being fair to yourself if you don't think about the options. . . . Yes, you will always be my daughter and I will always love you. I will accept your decision, but I will never tell you that the Marines are better for you than the Air Force. It's more than the fact that I was in the Air Force too. I have no doubt the Air Force will be everything you are seeking in the military, and more. . . . You will have something of an uphill fight in any service because you are a woman. Don't kid yourself. It isn't right but it is true. You will be a minority. People will respect you for your intelligence more in the Air Force. . . . I hope this isn't too late. I want you to stay in the Air Force. I love you. Dad

But deep down, in her gut, in her heart, Sarah knew the Marines was where she was supposed to be. Sarah felt *called* to be a Marine.

Sarah makes a point of recognizing that she didn't just rely on herself during that transition from Air Force to Marine Corps ROTC, though, as strong as she thought she was at 20 years old. She chose to also rely on the support of her closest friends, who heard her belabor the details of the choice over and over again and gave her good advice, who helped her train and prepare to become a Marine and helped her keep things light when the whole situation felt quite heavy at times. Also, Sarah's mentors at school were incredibly helpful, including the Marine Officer Instructor (MOI), a Major in the Marines, and the Assistant MOI, a Gunnery Sergeant, who believed in her, encouraged her, and trained her to succeed during the transition and beyond. Sarah was never left to do the work alone.

Here's the universal point: We've all been in a situation where we thought we might disappoint someone we love because of the choices we make about our particular path. Yet, to continue to live in a way that is out of alignment with who we are at our very core, can destroy us.

Connection, camaraderie, and community are vital, and every success story includes support from other people. All of Sarah's healthy transitions certainly involved the love and support of countless others.

Yet, we know we must also pay attention to our support from within, from our bodies. Not a visual of a youthful, fit, svelte body, but a supportive body that is an ally for action and balance; that is a resource of wisdom for us.

Although the power of intuition is something that's hard to describe with *words*, it's easy to *feel* within ourselves. We all know this when we say things like: "I just felt it in my gut" or "I knew it in my heart." Intuition requires awareness, that sometimes painful awareness, and we can choose to ignore our intuitions or we can choose to act on them.

How do we cultivate the habit of listening to our intuitive selves though? How do we listen to that intuition that lives in our hearts and our guts? We practice tuning in (in a variety of ways we'll share later), or we can try this: When you are about to make a decision, or potentially mistreat yourself or your body, pause, and ask yourself, "Is this how I would treat a good friend?" Our answer will come. And this is one very basic way to begin practicing awareness.

Our bodies are not machines, despite what all we hard-chargers think! Let's celebrate that we have a trusted friend (our body) to accompany us on our journey. Even when it supposedly "breaks," we can attempt to actually celebrate—or at least respect—the wisdom within our bodies, injuries and all, and be grateful for the messages that we receive from it and its ability to be our greatest ally because it is the house of our intuition. Our body's purpose is to faithfully support us. Our bodies help us find power *within* ourselves, not *over* ourselves.

Our bodies empower us to choose.

The second story we'd like to share with you in this introductory section of the book is about the sense of agency that can arise through choice-making, essentially about the power that making our own choices gives us. (Warning: this story includes some details about sexual assault.)

A second formative choice Sarah made happened a couple of years later in 2003. She was a Second Lieutenant in the U.S. Marine Corps (so the switch happened), and in the first week of The Basic School (TBS), she was doing her best to drink from the proverbial firehouse and absorb all the information they heard during orientation week.

One of the briefs they received was from the Judge Advocate General (the JAG). With sarcasm and disdain, the JAG warned a roomful of new officers about one of the most common "legal issues" they'd face while there: that they were likely going to rape one another at some point in their six-month training program. And it hit Sarah, "*What if the guy who raped me comes here and does that to someone else? I will never be able to live with myself.*"

And Sarah had a choice.

She *had* been raped, four months before, by a peer. And as the JAG told one particular story about a lieutenant raping another lieutenant there at TBS that sounded eerily similar to hers, she turned her head to the right and, in a room of more than two hundred lieutenants, locked eyes with the friend who she had called right after the assault. From across the room, her friend mouthed, "You have to tell."

Sarah mouthed back, "I know."

The day after she was raped, Sarah went to her MOI, the major who served as the leader of the Marine Corps-bound students within the Navy ROTC Battalion, and told him she didn't want to be a Marine anymore. She told him that she'd seen some things recently that made her believe she couldn't, shouldn't, and no longer wanted to be associated with the Marines. Sarah intended on telling her MOI that day that she had been raped. Like many survivors, she just couldn't find the words.

We know why victims do not want to tell because before *it* happens to you, you never think that it *could* happen to you, a strong, self-reliant person like you. But it did.

Sarah sucked it up though. She swallowed it and let it fester inside of her.

Then four months later, Sarah reported to Quantico Marine Corps Base as a Second Lieutenant. She completed Introductory Flight School (IFS) and then awaited her start of TBS, which is where this particular story began. That one day during orientation week of TBS, she sat in one of their classrooms and listened to the JAG describe other incidents of rape and sexual assault that had occurred between Marines at the training command. That JAG was flippant, sarcastic, and insincerely warned them about being careful not to get raped by each other.

So Sarah knew the military was notorious for mishandling rape cases.

Despite all of that, she felt like it was her duty to report it to possibly protect any potential future victims. Sarah was terrified the legal proceedings would take exactly the route that they did—isolation, fear, repeated questioning that left her feeling like the perpetrator, a victim of moral injury in addition to the initial trauma itself, with disruption of her training cycle and irrevocable damage to many of her personal relationships.

Although awful that it happened in the first place, and somehow even more awful going through the reporting process, Sarah says choosing to report the rape gave her a sense of agency.

Agency is that feeling of having a grip on your life, having a sense of influence or the feeling of being in charge of your own life. Yes, even in the midst of chaos.

It is not something Sarah would have chosen, of course—to have been raped—but given the option of staying in a black hole within herself or doing something that she felt could potentially protect a future victim, and something that gave her a sense of power of standing up for herself, Sarah still feels reporting was one of the best choices she ever made. As hard as it was and as damaging as it was to her personal and professional life in many ways, it was a choice that gave her power.

This is the universal point of this story: We all have these moments where we can choose to do the "hard" thing—often the "right" thing—*or* choose to keep our intuition, our wisdom, our character, or even our conviction to speak up on behalf of someone else buried.

Speaking up puts the dark thing into the light.

Even though it was around something negative, it made Sarah focus, it gave her purpose, and it made her connect to resources. As vulnerable as she already felt, it made her be more vulnerable in a way that guided her toward a deeper connection with others. Sarah formed deep friendships with those few who knew what she was going through. She sought professional counseling, confided in family, and began a journey of self-healing, introspection, and reflection that continues to this day. It fueled her ability to continue to sustainably serve even after she left active duty service.

Sarah's assailant, a peer, someone she knew, came into her home and attacked her.

He made a choice. Most of us have been hurt by something or someone who made a really bad choice.

Most of us have hurt ourselves at times, too.

Yet, we still have agency; we still have the power to choose again in the future.

Agency in the broader context of social science is the capacity of individuals to act independently and to make their own free choices. By contrast, structure is those factors of influence (such as social class, religion, gender, ethnicity, and customs) that determine or limit an agent and his or her decisions.

Therefore, in accepting that we all exist within a variety of structures—environmental, social, cultural, familial, ethnic, etc.—people continue to wrestle with when and how we have choice (or not) in our matters of living. How much do those structures and experiences limit us or not?

Viktor Frankl convincingly argues a variant of an oft-spoken line in yoga classes, "The space between stimulus and response is choice," or variations of that like, "You can choose to respond or react here." Pithy, perhaps, but Frankl better explains it by writing about his experience of many years spent in a Nazi concentration camp:

> The experiences of camp life show that man does have a choice of action. There were enough examples of a heroic nature, which proved that apathy could be overcome, irritability suppressed. Man can preserve a vestige of spiritual freedom, of independence of mind, even in such terrible conditions of psychic and physical stress. We who lived in concentration camps can remember the men who walked through the huts comforting others, giving away their last piece of bread. They may have been few in number, but they offer sufficient proof that everything can be taken from a man but one thing: the last of the human freedoms—to choose one's attitude in any given set of circumstances, to choose one's own way. And there were always choices to make.[1]

What a humbling comparison. That even in what is one of the direst of circumstances most of us could probably imagine, this man writes of having *choice*.

He goes on to say that those who essentially suffered with dignity, and who died with dignity, "bore witness to the fact that the last inner freedom cannot be lost."

It's not about emptying our heads or stopping our thoughts, but choosing which ones to pay attention to.

And there is dignity and meaning and value in the way in which we suffer. Have you admired someone who seemed to handle hit after hit that life threw at them without becoming bitter?

We have.

Suffering is unavoidable in our life, but our response to it is up to us. We can prepare for the hard times and tough transitions. That can change our mental health in powerful ways, allowing trauma to become fodder for post-traumatic growth.

The next sections of this text will discuss in detail how veterans can and are cultivating resilient traits in their own lives and in their communities. It can make a world of difference. Section two will focus on nervous system regulation, a key component of mental fitness and self-care. In section three, we will discuss the science of social support and identify ways veterans can and must work to build community post-service. In section four, we will discuss purposeful connection to action, sometimes referred to as spirituality. Finally, this book will link the science of resilience to a possible training method aimed at producing optimal mental health in our military veterans and at changing those complex suicide statistics.

NOTE

1. Here we quote from Viktor E. Frankl's book *Man's Search for Meaning*. Frankl was a prominent Viennese psychiatrist before World War II and is considered the father of logotherapy, who was uniquely able to observe the way both he and others in Auschwitz coped (or didn't) with the experience. He noticed that the men who comforted others survived the longest, proving that everything can be taken away from us except the ability to choose our attitude in any given set of circumstances. According to Frankl, the sort of person the concentration camp prisoner became was the result of an inner decision and not of camp influences alone. Frankl came to believe man's deepest desire is to search for meaning and purpose, and this is the founding theory of the therapeutic perspective known as logotherapy. Frankl, V. E. (2006). *Man's search for meaning.* Boston, MA: Beacon Press.

5

Military Mental Health

Kyle called her often late at night. Kate always had her cell phone on and close by in case he needed her. She usually slept with it by her pillow so she would be sure not to miss him. In truth, she knew it was very possible he would wind up in trouble somewhere.

Kate went through her days feeling tired a lot of the time.

Sometimes he would be drunk or high, wanting someone to tell him it was all going to turn out OK in the morning. One time he wanted her to go back to sleep but asked her to just leave the line open so he wouldn't be alone. She did.

Kate always did.

Part of her always expected a call from some emergency room or from his family sharing news of suicide or an overdose. When she left earlier that year, he had angrily thrown out the accusation that "Kate was leaving him for dead." She knew it was partly true, and she was terrified that she believed him, mostly because she just couldn't bear to turn off that phone.

This time the call was different. Kyle was on the line, speaking quietly. "Will you tell a Veterans Administration Social Worker that you will take possession of my guns? I need someone to vouch for my safety before they will let me go home from here." He was in Atlanta at an inpatient treatment facility.

Finally.

After years of battling some sort of mental health condition and accompanying self-medicating tendencies, he had checked himself in at the Department of Veterans Affairs (VA) hospital. He was tired and alone and afraid he might finally kill himself.

She packed her car and was on the way immediately, reading about protocols for visiting a patient in the lockdown ward by the afternoon. Kate followed the signs in the massive hospital complex to the inpatient mental health ward. A shiver went through her as she noticed the layers of locked doors and the signs warning visitors about coming in with certain items.

As the doors opened, a shrill buzzer sounded. She heard locks turning and for a long moment felt like running. This wasn't a world she was comfortable with—there were seriously mentally ill people beyond these doors!

What was she thinking coming here?

Divorced doesn't mean one doesn't care anymore.

Sometimes she wished it did.

Kate swallowed hard and stepped in and through the doors, no purse or pen. He knew she was on her way—he could always safely assume she would show up when asked, no matter what had happened the last time they saw one another.

He needed her. Or someone better at this than her.

Maybe that could happen here?

He was waiting for her past all the buzzers and locks. She saw him standing there in his brightly colored jumpsuit and tried to wrap her mind around where this had all wound up. He looked like a prisoner, and he sort of was one.

How could someone so beloved wind up here?

Was he the person she knew anymore?

Then he smiled. Kate recognized that wide smile and exhaled with relief.

*   *   *

Concern about military suicide rates and mental health seems to abound in popular media lately, but our understanding of those issues is limited and one-dimensional. Specifically, the current medical model asks us to talk about veteran mental health from a clinical standpoint.

Allow us to offer again an important disclaimer here—clinicians do valuable work, in particular the professionals who were deployed with the military to work in combat stress units. They offer an expert shoulder and save lives. In no way do we disparage their noble, effective work. However, any clinical practitioner will tell you that it can be tough to get military personnel in through their doors. For this reason, medical treatment can't remain the only conversation we are having about mental health in the military.

The medical model asks veterans struggling emotionally to label a problem and identify themselves as being in need of some sort of help. We use diagnostic labels like post-traumatic stress disorder (PTSD) or major depression to mark a veteran as permanently disabled; the Veterans Benefits Administration awards obscurely derived numeric ratings to men and women demonstrating symptoms. With a letter in the mail, one learns the exact percentage of "damaged" they are.

In some ways, this represents progress. Stress injury and depression are real, and pre-Vietnam, they were often discussed as nothing more than cowardice or moral failure. Moral injury is real, and we're only beginning to understand the complex ways it shows up in veterans' lives. In other ways, this readiness to label is a benevolent poison that tells veterans that their normal and adaptive symptoms after military service constitute permanent debilitation. It sets up stereotype expectations of brokenness in the public consciousness and asks the veteran to rely on therapeutic and pharmaceutical interventions to get "fixed." It talks about stress as a dangerous cause of injury rather than an opportunity to hone leadership, performance, and focus under fire. In fact, stress itself is meant to make us stronger and more resilient, so long as we put in place some key management tactics.

Studying mental health can be a complicated process, as symptoms manifest on multiple levels and vary greatly from one diagnosed patient to the next. Even the words we use to describe the symptoms vary greatly. Professionals discussing the same stress injury symptoms may refer to post-traumatic stress (PTS), the more stigmatizing PTSD, stress reaction, battle fatigue, operational stress, or shell shock. These trauma and stress disorder diagnoses are often accompanied by symptoms of depression in varying degrees of severity, and this co-occurrence may or may not be understood, recognized, and diagnosed.[1]

DEPRESSION

Depression is a diagnosis that covers a host of symptoms, categorized in *The Diagnostic and Statistical Manual of Mental Disorders* (*DSM-V*) by duration of symptom presence. Mild depression involves symptoms manifesting for more than four days, moderate depression involves symptoms for slightly longer periods, and major depression involves symptoms present almost every day for one month.

As with most psychological illnesses, symptoms manifest differently in every individual. Depression red flags include feelings of sadness, grief, worry, and tension and possible interference with daily activities as a result of these feelings. Some people experience loss of appetite or sex drive, while others go the opposite route and overeat or engage in promiscuous or risky sexual behavior.

Highly variant, depression is often ignored or even misdiagnosed, particularly in milder forms where treatment is most effective but diagnosis is hardest to pin down. Depression in some people looks a lot like stress injury, which is a normal and adaptive response to excess threats, whether those threats are present in the moment or are being reexperienced mentally in a flashback. In fact, stress and anxiety are symptoms of depression, and in some patients both conditions occur at the same time. The diagnoses are different, however.[2]

STRESS

Understanding stress injury requires understanding the absolutely normal way that our bodies respond to stressors. When something is at stake, we feel pressure to respond in some adaptive way. The brain tells our bodies to spring into action and sets in motion a chain of physical reactions. The human endocrine system is artfully wired to fire off a series of hormones whenever the brain registers something as threatening. Threats for a human are varied in terms of seriousness, but all trigger this exact same hormonal reaction in varying degrees of intensity.

The strongest reaction is the survival response known commonly as "fight or flight." This reaction gets the body ready for physical exertion, sending energy and resources to systems that are needed in a fight or a footrace. Heart rate increases, respiratory rate increases, and major muscles tense. Intense alertness may save a life in an immediate threat situation, but long term, an excessively firing fight-or-flight stress response causes problems. When stressed to this degree, the body shuts down nonessential systems to give energy and attention to major muscle groups, heart function, and breathing. If you are running from a lion, this physical state is very useful. However, the body also considers complicated thinking, muscle repair, reproductive functions, blood flow to fingers and toes, and digestion nonessential. Over time, problems arise as the body struggles to balance competing messages. Resources and blood flow to systems not necessary in extreme scenarios decrease. The immune, reproductive, and gastrointestinal systems are all examples. Ever get nauseous during an argument with your partner? Your body is responding to the prompting of stress hormones to stop digestion. We're not our brightest or most functional under fight-or-flight stress, which is dictated by simple stress response biology. It is the body adapting to threat as it knows to.

Cortisol and adrenaline course through the bloodstream of someone in severe distress, from the infant who can't make eye contact with a caregiver to the soldier experiencing his first firefight. This response is meant to help us fight or flee and operates in a negative feedback loop, meaning the response will shut itself off once the threat goes away. However, if a given threat is overly traumatic or simply goes on for too great a time, the stress response keeps firing, sending the entire nervous system into dysregulation. That little case of stomach butterflies may become a legitimate digestive ailment. That simple forgetfulness may become legitimate trouble focusing or memory problems. The elevated levels of cortisol and adrenaline present in the bloodstream of chronically stressed individuals directly impair the body's ability to shut down into restorative states.[3]

Our bodies release stress hormones in different amounts depending upon the severity of the stimulus. It is important to remember when we talk about stress that it isn't a simple "bad or good" binary. If the stimuli are not traumatic or severe, the body will respond in a couple of different ways to help us cope.

A particularly useful response is often referred to as the "stress challenge" response. Here, stress hormones (endorphins and adrenaline) are released at levels appropriate for promoting focus, energy, and drive to accomplish a task under pressure. Another common response is related to moderate release of stress hormones and an elevated level of oxytocin, the bonding hormone. This response is called the "tend and befriend" response, which involves people exhibiting extremely prosocial behavior when placed under some sort of pressure, particularly one related to a relationship. Here, we respond to our stress hormones and oxytocin by defending our loved ones or seeking help and connection from others. This response is what makes you want to call your best friend after a conflict at the office—you are seeking social support to cope with the pressure.

Biochemically, we grow from stress. The reason for this is an important hormone secreted during the stress response called dehydroepiandrosterone (DHEA). The job of this neurosteroid is to strengthen the brain after a stressful experience. This change can actually be seen in the frontal cortex when brain scans are conducted. Layers related to emotional control and logical reasoning thicken with exposure to DHEA over time. This growth and development process is highly adaptive if you think about it. We are meant to get stronger after facing pressure, to learn from growth opportunities, and to push our own limits.

Stress is a completely natural system response, and it has gotten a bad rap in medical circles. Eustress, or "good stress," drives performance and growth, and such pressures that are reasonable in duration and intensity help us become better, smarter, faster, and high-performing.

STRESS INJURIES

When a stressor is so severe that it triggers fight or flight and continues for too long without a recovery period, the body becomes injured and unbalanced. Our sympathetic nervous systems aggressively stay on, resulting in hypervigilance, insomnia, and a host of emotional regulation prob lems. A stress injury can make a person withdrawn, teary, or full of misplaced rage. Which symptoms manifest may depend only on what day of the week it is; they vary in and between individuals.

Interestingly, the vigilant and emotionally compartmentalized symptoms of stress injury double as essential survival skills in certain environments, which makes that injury useful (or even vital) in one setting and completely debilitating in another. A soldier's ability to dart eyes along a roadway in Iraq looking to swerve at any sign of debris or rock piles makes her a popular driver on convoys in-country. At home on the interstate, it just terrifies passengers.

Stress injury can certainly be a result of a one-time traumatic experience, but it can also be a result of chronically elevated hormone levels that cause the nervous system to remain in on-mode all the time. Anyone subjected to recurring stress stimuli over time is at risk of developing issues because their stress response will start staying on all the time. This abnormal stress reactivity and chronic stress response elevation becomes a stress injury, often called PTSD in clinical circles.

A fight or flight impulse that never goes away can wreak havoc on the human body. Researchers have studied long-term cognitive changes in soldiers and Marines post-deployment, looking at how stress reactions either enabled or impaired mission effectiveness. Their work found that in Iraq, the intensity made sense because the fast-moving landscape of the contemporary combat environment trains servicemembers to respond quickly and to spend most of their time in elevated states of alertness. Those states persisted up to two months after coming home, however. This is where the research team found the Marines struggling with focus, anxiety, and emotional outbursts.[4]

As previously mentioned, emotional reactivity is a hallmark symptom of a stress injury and can cause a vicious cycle of problems for sufferers as they create rifts in their support relationships. The reason for such reactivity is that long-term stress injury decreases something called working memory capacity. This higher-level brain function emotionally regulates us, allows us to bond and interact with one another socially, and makes advanced, intellectual activities such as Calculus possible. Losing working memory capacity can cause a host of emotional and behavioral problems and result in major issues with attention, focus, and regulation of responses.

In addition to being mental, stress injury symptoms can be physical. These may include some or all of the following: numbness in hands and feet, headaches, pain and inflammation, stomach problems, and high blood pressure. Though clinicians label it an injury, the body is only responding naturally to the messages cortisol and adrenaline are sending. The overactive stress response becomes ingrained in a patient with PTS symptoms, and a constant state of reactivity and hyper-arousal can begin to feel normal.

HOW LARGE IS THE MILITARY MENTAL HEALTH PROBLEM?

Statistics on PTS in veteran communities are uncertain, with estimates out of the Veterans Administration sitting at 15–50 percent. A RAND corporation study recently showed numbers hovering at about 20 percent. As one can derive from examining such wide reporting ranges, both stress injury and depression rates are largely unknown, and diagnosed depression is subject to semantic debate in the military community because symptom overlap between depressive conditions and stress injuries often leads to misdiagnosis.[5]

Here's the problem—when we talk about stress injury and depression as disorders, we give them an inaccurate air of permanence. Our body is meant to return to a balanced state of nervous system regulation, and PTS is a reversible injury at the mild and moderate levels of severity. The term "disorder" is a misnomer, applying only to the most severe cases as a chronic condition. Mild or moderate depression aren't permanent conditions either.

ARE ALL VETERANS STRUGGLING WITH DEPRESSION OR STRESS INJURY?

Contrary to some popular conceptions, stress injury is not an inevitable result of military service during wartime. In Israel, a country where every adult serves in the military for two years and war has been a common occurrence, rates of stress injury sit as low as 1 percent.

Many mental health issues are not causally linked to trauma. Misconceptions about "damaged war vets" actually contribute to stigma issues in veterans and to feelings that only certain people, with certain service histories, "rate" emotional struggles. In fact, combat exposure doesn't predict the likelihood that a veteran will commit suicide. Among younger veterans of Iraq and Afghanistan, the greatest predictor of suicide is not deployment, but rather a recent separation from service. Transition stress isolates, and that is more dangerous to mental health than a purposeful deployment with comrades. The reason for this lies in our human wiring. We are built to connect and commune with one another. When people cooperate and bond in close-knit groups, they increase levels of "happy hormones" like oxytocin and dopamine in their bloodstream. These hormones are in direct opposition to the stress hormones cortisol and adrenaline and have the opposite effect on the body. This relaxation response is triggered whenever we make a close connection, and loneliness and social rejection immediately set off the body's threat receptors.[6]

The veteran population in America is shrinking, and society's sense of purpose and connection to our wars of the last two decades is extremely limited. This all contributes powerfully to the higher rates of stress injury and depression we are seeing in young veterans. The issue seems to be one of alienation or isolation.

Treatment programs in the clinical mental health sector have been striving mightily over the last decade to stem the tide of service suicides. The Department of Defense and Veterans Administration have made combatting depression and stress injury a top priority, specifically because they are one of several known predictors of suicide.

We've done a great deal to try to understand the scope of the problem. Researchers have attacked the problem from different angles, looking at incidence rates to try to pin down a rate rather than a range. One telephone survey of 1,965 servicemembers who recently returned from Iraq highlighted the seriousness of depression prevalence; 14 percent met the criteria for PTS and major depression. A larger study the following year showed 36.9 percent of the 289,000 servicemembers surveyed had some sort of mental health diagnosis. Careful study of suicide risk in the military population compared to the general population shows that suicide risk is almost four times higher among young veterans than their non-serving peers, a difference made more statistically significant when analysis controls for age and time in service. Internationally, numbers indicate the same. A British study of recent veterans found the risk of suicide to be two to three times higher for military members leaving the service than the general population, with the year immediately following discharge being a particularly risky time.[7]

Beyond the numbers, researchers have asked veterans why they feel like they are struggling with mental wellness. A qualitative study published in the *American Journal of Public Health* aimed to probe more deeply the issue of post-discharge suicide risk in young veterans. Researchers conducted interviews of recently discharged troops diagnosed with depression and conducted general surveys of separating servicemembers who did not have a diagnosis. Their study demonstrated that major issues for veterans were reintegration into new roles and the loss of community that was felt when leaving the military. Veterans described a sense of burdensomeness and extreme disconnect from civilians. These feelings linked to a failed sense of belonging and desire for death. Follow-on studies focused specifically on female veterans, and they found that descriptions of symptoms and feelings of disconnect were markedly similar, though more pronounced and likely to be of greater severity. Some research has shown that transition can be even harder for subgroups of veterans who served on active duty as a numerical minority and who then have decreased access to support systems upon departure.[8]

For much of the last 18 years, the health community has asserted that if we know who is struggling, we can create specific programs to reach them and prevent suicide. This research is useful in providing roadmaps for providers hoping to target veterans by identifying variables and in expanding our scope of understanding concerning how to reach military veterans in culturally competent ways. Post-incident treatment must be part of the package as we work to make things better for veterans leaving the service, and we can always work on doing that better by expanding our reach and understanding. Here's the catch with such research and practice—the clinical recovery paradigm is limited. Veterans are not excited about embracing patient identities and accepting diagnoses. We'd rather talk training for performance than recovery from a wound. The challenge for health professionals looking to stem the tide of service suicides and to improve quality of life for veterans lies in shifting from a focus on problems toward a focus on capacity-building. In this space, we may have a massive opportunity to make a positive impact.

NOTES

1. There have been outstanding analyses of the problems with mental health diagnoses in military personnel by former service physicians. Stress injury looks like depression, and the symptoms work well in an intense environment. In many ways, these mental health "problems" are absolutely adaptive. Hoge, C. W. (2010). *Once a warrior, always a warrior* (1st ed.). Guilford, CT: Lyons Press; Hoge, C. W., & Castro, C. A. (2012). Preventing suicides in U.S. service members and veterans. *Journal of American Medical Association, 308*(7), 671–672.

2. Understanding the ways in which depression and stress injuries are categorized in the clinical setting is complicated, as symptoms vary between patients, and the conditions often either co-occur or look markedly similar. Bossarte, R. M. (Ed.). (2013). *Veterans suicide: A public health imperative* (1st ed.). Washington, D.C.: American Public Health Association; Calhoun, P. S., Hertzberg, J. S., Kirby, A. C., Dennis, M. F., Hair, L. P., Dedert, E. A., & Beckham, J. C. (2012). The effect of draft DSM-V criteria on posttraumatic stress disorder prevalence. *Depression & Anxiety, 29*(12), 1032–1042; American Psychiatric Association. *Diagnostic and statistical manual of mental disorders: DSM-5.* (2013). Washington, D.C.: American Psychiatric Association.

3. The human stress response is a normal adaptation meant to keep us safe in reaction to a perceived threat. It only becomes a health problem when it doesn't shut off. This can occur when a stressor is so traumatic that the brain keeps reexperiencing it or when stressors are chronic. Romas, J. A., & Sharma, M. (2010). *Practical stress management: A comprehensive workbook for promoting health and managing change through stress reduction* (5th ed.). San Francisco, CA: Benjamin Cummings; Seaward, B. (2019). *Managing stress: Principles and strategies for health and well-being.* Sudbury, MA: Jones and Bartlett.

4. Studies on the impact of stress show that unchecked fight- or flight-level responses impair us on both physiological and neurological levels. Interestingly, this can be reversed by using relaxation techniques to activate the parasympathetic nervous system and calm the stress response. That is why we often hear that taking time to relax can make us mentally sharper; it actually changes our brain tissue! Jha, A. P., & Kiyonaga, A. (2010). Working-memory-triggered dynamic adjustments in cognitive control. *Journal of Experimental Psychology: Learning, Memory, and Cognition, 36*(4), 1036–1042; Jha, A. P., Stanley, E. A., Kiyonaga, A., Wong, L., & Gelfand, L. (2010). Examining the protective effects of mindfulness training on working memory capacity and affective experience. *Emotion, 10*(1), 54–64.

5. We don't really know how many veterans are suffering from stress injuries because they are notoriously misunderstood, misdiagnosed, and stigmatized. Ranges vary from 15 to 50 percent depending on the source. Acosta, J., Reynolds, K., Gillen, E. M., Feeney, K. C., Farmer, C. M., & Weinick, R. M. (2014). *The RAND online measure repository for evaluating psychological health and traumatic brain injury programs.* Washington, D.C.: RAND Corporation; Coughlin, S. S. (Ed.). (2012). *Posttraumatic stress disorder and chronic health conditions* (1st ed.). Washington, D.C.: American Public Health Association; Department of Veterans Affairs. *Mental health and Military Sexual Trauma.* Accessed February 19, 2020, Available at http://www.mentalhealth.va.gov/msthome.asp

6. Cooperating socially and experiencing social support in a warm community are adaptive behaviors for which we are wired. Studies have shown that close networks in close communities increase life expectancy by as much as 7.5 years, and people without strong social networks fare worse when recovering from injury or surgery. To lose community is the ultimate stressor for a brain wired for connection, and that is exactly what veterans experience when they leave the military and return to a civilian world that may no longer feel like home. Transition, then, becomes a traumatic stressor. Junger, S. (2016). *Tribe: On homecoming and belonging.* New York, NY: Hachette; Thomas, K. H., Haring, E., McDaniel, J. T., Fletcher, K., Albright, D. L., & Brandley, E. (2019). Belonging and support for women veterans. In Thomas, K. H. & Hunter, K. (Eds.), *Invisible veterans: What happens when service women become civilians again* (pp. 57–68). Santa Barbara, CA: ABC-CLIO/Praeger Publishing.

7. Research into stress injury and depression prevalence has identified some of the issues the services face with these mental health conditions as they relate to combat deployments. Interestingly, deploying doesn't make problems more likely than remaining in garrison. Ilgen, M. A., McCarthy, J. F., Ignacio, R. V., Bohnert,

A. B., Valenstein, M., Blow, F. C., & Katz, I. R. (2012). Psychopathology, Iraq and Afghanistan service, and suicide among Veterans Health Administration patients. *Journal of Consulting and Clinical Psychology, 80*(3), 323–330; Seal, K. H., Metzler, T. J., Gima, K. S., Bertenthal, D., Maguen, S., & Marmar, C. R. (2009). Trends and risk factors for mental health diagnoses among Iraq and Afghanistan veterans using Department of Veterans Affairs health care, 2002–2008. *American Journal of Public Health, 99*(9), 1651–1658; Tanielan, T., & Jaycox, L. H. (2008). *Invisible wounds of war: Psychological and cognitive injuries, their consequences, and services to assist recovery.* Washington, D.C.: RAND Corporation.

8. Qualitative studies that ask in-depth questions often find that military personnel and veterans feel deeply alienated from nonveterans. Albright, D. L., Fletcher, K., Thomas, K. H., O'Brien, M., & Godfrey, K. (2018). Older military veterans. In Castro, C. & Weiss, E. (Eds.), *American military life in the 21st century: Social, cultural, economic issues and trends* (pp. 546–558). Santa Barbara, CA: ABC-CLIO/Praeger Publishing; Brenner, L. A., & Barnes, S. M. (2012). Facilitating treatment engagement during high-risk transition periods: A potential suicide prevention strategy. *American Journal of Public Health, 102*, S12–S14; Gutierrez, P. M., Brenner, L. A., Rings, J. A., Devore, M. D., Kelly, P. J., Staves, P. J., & Kaplan, M. S. (2013). A qualitative description of female veterans' deployment-related experiences and potential suicide risk factors. *Journal of Clinical Psychology, 69*(9), 923–935; Seamone, E. R., Thomas, K. H., & Albright, D. L. (2018). Incarcerated veterans. In Church, W. (Ed.), *Serving the stigmatized: Working within the incarcerated environment* (pp. 307–332). Cary, NC: Oxford University Press; Thomas, K. H. (2019). The two liminalities of war. In Carson, T. (Ed.), *Understanding liminality* (pp. 72–83). Cambridge, UK: Lutterworth Press.

SECTION SUMMARY

Imagine that you're out playing a game of afternoon football and you tear your ACL. No doctor would simply give you a diagnosis and some medications and then send you on your way. Instead, you'd likely have surgery followed by regular physical therapy visits. You'd also learn more effective warm-ups and conditioning and use them on a regular basis to stay injury-free in the future.

The same principles apply for recovery from post-traumatic stress injuries, sometimes called post-traumatic stress disorder (PTS/PTSD). With optimal behavioral health practices, it is possible to experience either total healing or marked improvement for mild to moderate stress injuries.

The idea that PTSD is an unalterable lifetime sentence is neurologically untrue.

Stress Injuries versus PTSD

Stress injuries are very natural responses to unusual situations and exist along a spectrum. Whether you've experienced a single traumatic event or multiple stressors over a long period of time, your body likely responded in a totally appropriate way by adapting to the threat. Your nervous system kicked into high gear—your body and brain woke up and went into overdrive.

Your response was vital to navigating a stressful or dangerous situation well. However, now that imminent danger is past, your stress response may still activate out of context. When this happens, empathy may disappear, your focus may degrade, and you may struggle to make logical decisions.

It's true that severe stress injury (also known as PTSD) is a complicated disorder. However, health-care practitioners often apply the "chronic" label to mild or moderate stress injuries—which are 100 percent recoverable. This label can be psychologically deadly—sapping resilient people of the agency they need to learn and apply tools to quickly de-escalate the body's and brain's response to perceived threats.

The truth is that PTSD is not everyone's stress injury. A misdiagnosis suggests irrecoverable brokenness and can layer on a host of additional anxieties and worries.

Road to Recovery

One of the most empowering first steps you can take toward recovery is to seek out information about stress physiology—work to understand what is happening in your body.

Self-education is an incredibly empowering step. You'll discover that your out-of-context responses are natural, and you'll simultaneously find ways to calm your body and mind through a variety of self-care practices.

When you put these tools into practice on a daily basis, your body and brain will respond in some really interesting ways. Your neurons will fire differently; you'll shrink the amygdala (the part of your brain that activates the fight or flight response)—your brain will literally start to look different. Stress hormones will drop, too.

Not only will your body and mind change, but so will your behavior. You'll find that you're better able to handle a disagreement with your partner. You'll be able to focus better and exist with more empathy. Of course, you're still human. Your stress response will still fire (as it should). But by practicing effective self-care, you can begin to respond to others in a more deliberate way.

But What If My Stress Injury Is Severe?

Some people experience permanent changes to their brains. If your injury co-occurs with a traumatic brain injury, depression, or an anxiety disorder, that is totally normal, but incredibly challenging. When you have a major stress injury and you're dealing with a chronic condition, the symptoms can be extremely debilitating.

The symptoms of severe stress injuries can be improved upon, but—much like a bad back injury—you may need to accept that your condition will need to be managed for many years to come.

For severe stress injury, you will need highly individualized clinical help. Seek medical guidance and talk to your clinician about your specific stress injury and wellness techniques.

SECTION 2

Self-Care

6

Regulating the Nervous System for Mental Fitness

Legendary U.S. Marine Corps Gen. James "Mad Dog" Mattis once said, "The most important six inches on the battlefield is between your ears."

Servicemembers who are deployed during today's complex conflicts have a special appreciation for Mattis' assertion that the mind matters most.

THE CHALLENGE

In an era where the military is heavily involved in both combat operations and nation-building, troops are often expected to simultaneously sustain focus; make nuanced, split-second decisions about the use of force; *and* reach back into their memories to draw on their training during high-stress situations. Then we are expected to return home and shift seamlessly into a civilian life with its own stressors and fast pace.

These efforts and both settings require a high frontal cortex functional capacity. The frontal cortex helps us with both emotional regulation (being able to think and not just react) and upper level cognition (focus). These brain functions comprise our working memory capacity, and interestingly, we can improve that capacity with the use of some well-studied, relatively simple exercises.

Unfortunately, although the military emphasizes the importance of physical training and does a wonderful job creating developmental stress opportunities, it doesn't do a great job of training servicemembers to rest or do the restorative practices needed to maximize the mind's growth opportunities. When we speak about self-care, we are speaking more about nervous system regulation done intentionally.

Restorative practices move our bodies to a rested state between action and sleep. These practices matter because they increase our physical and mental performance, which are important both in and out of the military. The same things that make you a better warrior can also make you a better parent, partner, employee, and friend.

WHY DOES MENTAL FITNESS TRAINING MATTER?

For active duty servicemembers and veterans alike, mental fitness training should include stressors alongside very intentional mental recovery time. When both are combined, physical and mental performance increase, clarity of thought improves, and you're able to slow your reaction times in the right contexts.

Self-care is a word in vogue today, but few people actually practice it. We live amidst an epidemic of chronic overstimulation and tend to embrace treatment of the health issues that come along with that rather than do the harder, slower work of bringing our nervous systems back into a regulated state.

When we talk about caring for our physical body, we often emphasize movement and challenge. In actuality, balance is one of the most important things a person can plan into a training calendar. The physical practices that offer us stress reduction and a return to homeostatic balance are beneficial in a myriad of ways. Balanced physical self-care with a keen focus on regulating an overstimulated nervous system must become priorities to anyone looking to cultivate resilience. That restorative practice is what allows stress to grow the brain.

Here's the good news—there is more than one way to find restorative states. You have the freedom to figure out which activities work best for your personality, resources, and preferences. It is beyond the scope of this book to outline every health practice available to promote a resilient physical state, and we will endeavor simply to share the merit of self-care in whatever form feels most appealing to the individual.

Trying out mindful movement practices and learning from the pros who teach them is one of our favorite hobbies. For the authors, the most relaxing physical practice available changes based on what's happening in their daily livees. There have been times when the answer was trail running, yoga, swimming, or rowing. Healthy practices are not abusive. When it is a balancing activity, you'll feel yourself exerting but peaceful. You will sleep a bit better. You may notice your mind steady. You may pay attention to your body in a new way. Such training involves purposeful movement that brings attentive focus to the physical body and the racing mind. This attention trains the body in both challenging and balanced fashion, while carving in space for activation of the parasympathetic nervous system. The parasympathetic nervous system activates when the body is in a peaceful, flow state. It is here that the body restores and improves, and hormone levels in the blood go back to their optimal levels.

Mindful movement is a unique way to build mental toughness; it creates opportunities for mastery experience and a platform from which to build physical stability. Interestingly, most of us are not physically stable without very intentionally working to become so. We sit too much and slouch a bit, and we create muscular imbalances that we don't notice because we often zip through our days without paying attention to present-tense sensations in our tissues.

As discussed in an earlier chapter, the stress response is a completely natural phenomenon, and the human body operates intelligently to produce appropriate reactions to life's surprises. Upon registering some sort of threat, the brain sends hormonal signals to the adrenal glands, which secrete cortisol and adrenaline to empower the body to handle it. In a healthy negative feedback system, the cortisol signals the hypothalamus to shut down the response, provided the threat has disappeared. This stress response happens at an intensity level in relation to the threat. It is instinctual and animal and is necessary for performance, self-preservation, and survival.

Everyone's response to stimuli differs, and what is stimulating to one person biochemically may not be to another. That doesn't mean our systems aren't registering the stimulation, however. The problem with the human stress response does not become apparent until the stress becomes chronic, and the bloodstream contains too much cortisol. Chronic stress occurs when the brain's hypothalamus refuses to shut off the chemical signals it is sending because it still perceives a problem. In our modern society with constantly ringing phones, troubled interpersonal relationships, and an ever-increasing pace enabled by technology, chronic stress is rampant.

When the body's stress response is constantly firing, blood cortisol levels are too high and inflammatory proteins become more present in the bloodstream. A host of illnesses and inflammatory conditions have been related to this chemical imbalance. The body's immune system becomes overactive and confused by the aberrant proteins. Unsure which foreign bodies to attack, autoimmune illnesses like rheumatoid arthritis and allergies become real health issues. Unchecked, unacknowledged stress is a killer in too many ways to count. Chronic stress has been linked to a host of physical maladies, including abdominal weight gain, cancer, gastrointestinal illnesses, depression, and chronic pain.[1]

We can't always prevent surprises that send our bodies into reaction mode, but we can prepare them for stress and adopt a positive outlook toward challenge, in general. Consider self-care preventive training because planning intentional downtime for the nervous system truly is!

Think about the last time you experienced stress. Maybe it was being stuck behind a slow driver in traffic or gearing up for a mandatory run with a wicked hangover. Maybe it was being in a firefight or being lost somewhere. Here's a snapshot of what happens in your body in those scenarios: Your brain operates in an active state, indicated by what researchers call Beta waves. This is a high-functioning mental space. As the stress is registered by your brain, a chain reaction fires. Your body releases cortisol (a stress hormone), adrenaline, and a host of other chemicals to help you cope. It also releases a hormone called DHEA into your bloodstream.

DHEA's entire role is to help your brain grow from the stressor you just survived. The hormone increases synaptic firing and neural connectivity (you'll think faster) and increases working memory capacity (emotional regulation and focus). DHEA is what makes stressful experiences worth your time, *but there's a catch*: although the hormone is released when your body or brain are stressed, it only does its work during recovery time—when your body and brain consciously downshift.

One of the best validated ways to move your brain to this state is through mindfulness-based stress reduction, or—as it is more commonly known—meditation.

Meditation takes your brain from Beta state (alert, on guard) to Theta space (at rest, but aware). When you sleep, your brain produces Delta waves (deep, dreamless sleep).

Meditation is one of the fastest ways to give your mind and body the space they need to turn stress into strength. Even if you only dedicate 15 minutes each day to it, you're likely to see dramatic changes in your ability to focus and regulate emotions within a week or two of practice.

Every hurdle you jump over and every stress or trigger you encounter becomes more useful if you carve out recovery time. Meditation is performance enhancement—it trains us for mental fitness.

Health is a term commercially co-opted. Rarely do we discuss healthy practices as interrelated, highly personalized techniques for bringing base-level balance to a person. We often talk about ideal aesthetics or extreme performance instead. In reality, simple things are actually important health practices. For example, sitting still out in nature activates the body's relaxation response and creates space for cognitive recovery and growth.

The types of practices that create bodily strength and balance are very different from those touted to meet an appearance metric. These focused practices are not additional stressors on the body, but rather, they provide physical buttress and support that both regulate the nervous system and build resilience. Training still means pushing the envelope to promote growth, but to build resilience and healthy practices that lower stress, regulate the nervous system, and bring attention to muscular imbalances are the building blocks of a self-care regimen.

For many, it can be fascinating to learn about the evidence basis for meditation and yoga that are termed as self-care modalities. There are many definitions and branded phrases to describe the form of therapeutic yoga used to treat patients. Typically, yoga interventions involve still, seated meditation; physical movements of varying difficulty levels; and instructional seminars on individual peace, spirituality, and stress management.

Yoga links breath to bodily movement in poses meant to create both strength and flexibility. It can be practiced in a variety of styles, but it always involves an element of focused attention on breath and body. In a society where we are often moving too fast, yoga asks us to do more than simply exercise; it asks us to slow down and pay attention, activating our parasympathetic nervous system and giving our tissues and minds space to recharge.

One of the best reasons to give yoga a try as a self-care modality is that science supports its usefulness. The practice of yoga has been successful in reducing the immediate and chronic effects of stress and enhancing overall health, and it offers physical and emotional benefits that may assist in the prevention and treatment of serious illness. The worth of mindful movement has been tested in cancer patients, the elderly, the depressed, and the hyperactive.

In particular, yoga does great things for mental well-being. A study published in the *Journal of Cognitive Behavioral Therapy* charted the self-reported quality of life improvements in two groups of physically healthy participants currently participating in cognitive behavioral therapy (CBT) for stress-related anxiety. The intervention group continued the therapy and participated in an intervention based on meditation and physical yoga. The control group continued their regimen of CBT alone. The group incorporating yoga into their routine reported significantly higher quality of life indicators.

Chronic pain has been successfully treated with yoga in several studies. The *Clinical Journal of Pain* follows closely interventions of a complementary and alternative nature, and it has published in 2011 the latest results from a long-term study on military veterans. Veterans with nonmalignant pain undertaking a yoga practice and meditation course reported reduced severity of their pain. Another study in Washington, D.C., in 2014 found that not only could six weeks of yoga reduce patients' pain, it could also reduce blood cortisol levels.

Distress compromises the immune system because fight or flight views sending energy to stave off illness as nonessential. Long-term, chronic stress causes a host of problems for people trying to stay healthy because their T-cells are under-resourced and unable to do their jobs! Immuno function in particular has been shown to improve with yoga-based intervention. A study among college-aged females practicing for 12 weeks showed functionality improvements at the middle and study-completion testing points.[2]

Taking care of our physical body goes a long way toward readying us to deal with a crisis when it erupts. Managing stress, eating well, and moving are all important. Intentionally down-regulating the nervous system on a daily basis is an essential component of a self-care routine. Because our physical bodies are linked to our mental states, taking care of the body takes care of the mind. Rates of depression, anxiety, stress, and stress-related health problems all go down when we become active.[3]

NOTES

1. Health problems are an undeniable result of chronic stress, which decreases a person's resilience. Larkin, K. T. (2005). *Stress and hypertension: Examining the relation between psychological stress and high blood pressure.* New Haven, CT: Yale University Press; Romas, J., & Sharma, M. (2010). *Practical stress management* (5th ed.). San Francisco, CA: Benjamin Cummings; Seaward, Brian. (2010). *Managing stress* (7th ed.). Burlington, MA: Jones and Bartlett.

2. The physical practice of yoga has been proven to offer the benefit of a fitness modality with both the stress relief of prayer and quiet contemplation. Stress-related illness is a modern epidemic. According to the American Medical Association, three out of every four doctors' visits involve illnesses related to chronic stress. To complement traditional treatments, the utilization of the practice of yoga offers promise. Some Department of Veterans Affairs (VA) hospitals conduct yoga and meditation seminars for patients suffering from a host of maladies. Evans, S., Tsao, J. C. I., Sternlieb, B., & Zeltzer, L. K. (2009). Using the biopsychosocial model to understand the health benefits of yoga. *Journal of Complementary & Integrative Medicine, 6*(1), 1–22; Farhi, D. (2000). *Yoga mind, body, and spirit* (1st ed.). New York, NY: Holt; Granath, J., & Ingvarsson, S. (2006). Stress management: A randomized study of cognitive behavioural therapy and yoga. *Cognitive Behavior Therapy, 35*(1), 3–10; Smeeding, S., Bradshaw, D. H., Kumpfer, K. L., Trevithick, S., & Stoddard, G. J. (2011). Outcome evaluation of the Veterans Affairs Salt Lake City Integrative Health Clinic for chronic

nonmalignant pain. *The Clinical Journal of Pain, 27,* 146–155; Thomas, K. H., & Plummer Taylor, S. (2015). Bulletproofing the psyche: Mindfulness interventions in the training environment to improve resilience in the military and veteran communities. *Advances in Social Work, 16*(2), 312–322.

3 Healthy behaviors are linked to better mental health status. In the diet, this means limiting alcohol and eating clean foods. Physically, this means adopting balanced activity programs and carving space for nervous system regulation. Harrington, A. (2008). *The cure within: a history of mind-body medicine.* New York, NY: WW Norton & Company; Koenig, H. G. (Ed.). (1998). *Handbook of religion and mental health.* West Conshohocken, PA: Elsevier; Thomas, K. H. (2017, November). *Bulletproofing the Psyche* for TEDx. Accessed July 6, 2020, Available at https://www.ted.com/talks/kate_thomas_bulletproofing_the_psyche

7

Practicing Mindfulness

Because yoga is one form of a mindfulness-based practice that is so much more than an avenue to self-comfort, because it is a truly evidence-based form of self-care, addressing it in more details is vital in the suicide prevention landscape.

Sarah initially hated yoga. Several friends and co-workers suggested it to her throughout the years, but it didn't "click" for her until she was in a time of complete crisis. Since then, learning more about the proven benefits of it has helped her maintain her practice as the seasons of her life have continued to change. In retrospect, the tipping point was when she first felt the initial awareness of her own mind-body connection via yoga, which then gave her a sense of power and agency in situations in which she previously felt out of control. She felt she was able to *sense* what was actually happening within her being, psyche, heart, and soul, and subsequently, she felt equipped to respond to situations versus react one breath at a time. Sarah's breath gave her a sense of choice, and her breath was refined and enhanced via a regular yoga practice.

The root of the words *inspire, aspire,* and *expire* is *spirare* from the Latin word meaning to breathe. As we strive to inspire others, we fill them with fire, or we hope they'll feel a "fire in their belly" or a "fire in their hearts," and fire requires oxygen, or breath. As we aspire to do anything, we must breathe life into it. And when we die, we exhale; we release our last breath.

Breathwork, in addition to movement and gently focused attention, is one key component of yoga. Breathwork refers to many forms of conscious alteration of breathing. A simple example is intentionally connecting the inhale and exhale in some measured way or energetically charging and discharging by using the breath to do so, two methods often used within psychotherapy, yoga, meditation, or other healing modalities. Teaching and practicing breathwork is a key component of our professional work and personal practices not only because we have experienced the benefits firsthand but also because research such as a Harvard Medical School study from 2013 showed that simply knowing breath-management techniques and having a better understanding and awareness of stress can help build resilience.[1]

The term *meditation,* which is often a component of yoga associated with cultivated, focused attention, also refers to a broad variety of practices (much like the term *sports*) that includes techniques designed to promote relaxation; build internal energy or life force; guide prayer and focus; and develop compassion, love, and patience.

Yoga can be used to direct and enhance the body's energy and aid in the release of old emotions, often leading to a sense of renewal, healing, or rejuvenation. In a physical sense, yoga is the union of breath and movement to build well-being. Per research, breathwork, meditation, and yoga are the three main components of "mindfulness practices" that light up the compassion center of our brains and helps us form new neural pathways; these practices enhance our physical balance, our endocrine balance, and nervous system balance. Day in, day out, we live with stress, and that's actually okay. We *do* require stress to survive, and in many instances (as previously mentioned) to even grow stronger.

What matters is how stress affects our nervous system and how we process it emotionally based on how we perceive its impact. So mindset is pretty important! But it can't be entirely impacted by conscious choice; *we've got to rewire a stress- or trauma-ravaged brain and nervous system to equip us to make those mindset and action choices.* We'll never eliminate stress completely; that is not the aim. The aim is to improve our relationship with feelings of stress, anxiety, and depression, ultimately learning to tolerate distress—not to obsess over our problems to the point that we fuse with them, nor to be in such denial that we never even get the opportunity to change or heal what needs changing or healing. Maybe this is the other side of the coin for those of us who are goal-oriented and want to jump right to the place where we eliminate symptoms. Focusing solely on eliminating symptoms can get us either stuck in them or magnify them, though. There's a sweet spot, a middle ground, somewhere in between those two extremes that regular mindfulness practices, like breathwork exercises, gives us access to.

So, the aim is to be dynamic and responsive, not stagnant and reactive. We must surf the waves, not strive to make them stop. And we need to know how to do that.

Every day, nearly twenty veterans die from suicide. Every day, too many veterans feel separate, alone, misunderstood, and hardened to the world. And these mindfulness practices can help veterans stop ending their own lives. These tools are not nice-to-haves; they are lifesavers!

Maybe veterans have more experience with a particular type of pain and trauma than the average American, but we *all* have pain and trauma; we all have battle zones such as divorce, illness, loss of a loved one, financial hardship, chronic business, and times when we feel like we have control over nothing.

So, how can pain be a teacher and not an enemy? We need to think of stress, trauma, and injury less as needs for treatment and more as opportunities for training. Because, let's be serious, the veteran mindset is not one that responds well to victimization or pathologizing of their problems. We need to be more proactive. We need to help soldiers, sailors, airmen, and Marines up-armor ahead of time with tools they can take with them anywhere in any situation. All post-traumatic stress (PTS) does *not* come just from combat. It comes from other "battlefields" too. Even for those in treatment settings, if we can design it to be more like training so we can destigmatize health practices to be presented as mindfulness and resilience-building tool sets that "bulletproof" our brains, we'll be speaking the language of resiliency, of awareness, of agency, of connection, and ultimately of *choice*.

What if military personnel were being proactively taught to respect the waves of anxiety, depression, and stress that surely come as a survivor of chaos, various traumas, or combat just as a surfer is taught to respect the strong waves of the ocean? To revere them, train for them, and honor their wisdom? What if we could be helped to understand things that way? What if our warriors today can cultivate that understanding? To be able to respect and honor our minds and bodies instead of feeling betrayed by them is a game changer that mindfulness fuels.

Intuition, agency, connection, and awareness are all choices. They don't just happen. They can be practiced and improved. We can choose to act, even little bits at a time, and we can choose to connect, one breath at a time. It is a practice in and of itself that improves with time and attention to it.

We'd like to offer you a way to connect now, with some simple and powerful breathwork. This is just one type of breathwork we frequently use with our clients and students, as well as in our daily practices, and it is called "square breath." It is known to calm our nervous system and get us "grounded" and connected to our bodies. It can sometimes produce a feeling of "balance" as well.

Who knew there were so many ways to breathe? This is just one. Here we go.

Sit somewhere comfortable, either on the ground or in a chair. If in a chair, if possible, place both feet on the floor and sit up straight, but not rigid. To start, close your mouth gently and keep your jaw relaxed while you begin to inhale and exhale just through your nose. Do that a few times, then begin square breath: inhale as you count to four, then pause and hold your breath in (but stay relaxed in the face, jaw, and shoulders in particular!) for a count of four, then exhale to a count of four, and then pause and hold the breath out for a count of four. So it's inhale for four, hold the breath in for four, exhale for four, hold the breath out for four. Start by practicing five rounds of that. Increase this gradually as you develop your breathing practice. Then give yourself a minute or two to sit quietly afterward, simply breathing in whatever way feels comfortable.

Even when all else is raging around us, swirling in our respective battle zones, the one thing we can always *choose* is our breath. It changes our brains, our bodies, and our hearts. It gives us access to somatically based knowledge that can be incredibly helpful in personal and professional settings. It's always ours; it's personal. No one can ever touch it. It's the one thing we all do all the time whether we consciously think about it or not. It unites us to our strongest self and helps us connect to others. Breath steadies the pace of life and creates space for reflection—*breath makes space for choice.*

Our lives begin and end with breath, and in the space in between, intentional breath helps us make intentional choices.

So, although Sarah began sporadically practicing yoga in the early 2000s in college to deal with overtraining injuries from soccer and Air Force Reserve Officer Training Corps (ROTC), it held no special importance to her beyond creative cross-training until she was in the midst of her second deployment in Iraq. Honestly, she'd barely done yoga before she went to Iraq; she didn't even really like it. Sarah was the person who often left in the middle of class or walked out during *savasana* (final resting pose), but she'd heard yoga was good for you, so she kept trying it sporadically. Sarah worked with a Marine who was bold enough to keep telling her, "Ma'am, you need this," and he gave her one of his yoga DVDs during her first deployment. She was willing to take a risk and give it a try again.

Then in Iraq, without even consciously processing the higher transformation that was taking place within her, when Sarah was emotionally distraught, yoga gave her a sense of clarity. The simple, basic union of breath and movement made space for the two most important things in her life—her choice and her sense of heart and soul.

Somehow, in a body experiencing the very physical effects of depression, and other severe physical injuries, when she practiced yoga, she noticed less pain. Somehow, in a world that felt like 24/7 chaos, like a battle zone at all times, the mat gave her an anchor point with which to align.

Thank goodness for that 3' x 6' floor space because it was where Sarah could simply breathe without suffocating. She would roll off her bed onto her yoga mat and things would change. She would align. She could breathe. If she was lucky, things would release. She would stretch, and then she would breathe, and then she'd go for a run and feel free.

Stretch.
Breathe.
Move.
Stretch.
Breathe. Move . . . Breathe. Connect.

If Sarah was lucky, she would connect first to something beyond herself, then to those around her; it meant she was alive. She would repeat to herself, "I'm breathing. I'm alive. I'm breathing. I'm alive." It was that simple for Sarah at that point in her life. To breathe meant to be alive, and to be alive meant to believe in more.

She knew she certainly was not the only one going through what she was going through. She was not the first or last lost soul who found herself in a battle zone. When Sarah realized that—that her lack of "specialness" was actually a blessing in this case and that her baggage wasn't a burden, but touchstones for growth—the accessibility to healing became greater, deeper, and more diverse.

Sarah was a hardcore yoga skeptic, turned yoga student, turned yoga teacher. It's been quite the evolution from her "*it's not worth exercising unless it kicks my butt*" days to where she is now (more than twenty years later). She admits that she is still both a student and a teacher at all times. She is a recovering perfectionist with plenty of interesting baggage with which to work. Again, realizing that she is not special in that regard—that we've all got baggage, insecurities, and (mental and physical) injuries—has helped her immensely. Yoga, for all its feel-good niceties, bendiness, and fit bodies, isn't all sunshine and butterflies all the time. Yoga can absolutely bring your baggage up too. Yoga can create the refining fires that we need to walk through when we start to notice and feel things that we've buried or avoided for so long. The question is, How do you meet the challenge of the fire without getting burned up? You do so by keeping your nervous system consistently regulated or dedicating extra time to downregulate during especially stressful times.

Yet, sometimes even a disciplined dedication to mindfulness can feel like a source of stress if we let it. Thus, these three simple yet powerful reminders help Sarah work through, for example, a painful and frustrating yoga class. We hope they help you, too:

1. **It's all about the breath.** Yes, it's that simple. Thank goodness it is. You can take heart in knowing that even if you just sit there without touching your nose to your toes, if you are breathing mindfully, then you are doing something good for yourself.

2. **Modifying doesn't equal cheating.** There are lots of yoga theories out there, some of which think that using props is a crutch. We strongly disagree. If you need to modify a posture by throwing a block under your booty or a strap around your foot so you can enjoy the intended opening and keep your breath smooth at the same time, great, do it. Modifying without props by utilizing the diversity of our own body is another way to tangibly meet ourselves where we are.

3. **This is your healing work.** Injuries do not have to be lifelong burdens sent to punish you. Regardless of your faith background, this general lesson is applicable across many areas of life. Essentially, as you heal, you make space for others to heal; as you take care of yourself, you give permission to others to do so, as well. And we must change within before we can expect to change the world.

Look, Sarah can't do forearm stand; can't do sundial; can't do cow face pose; she most certainly cannot sit in full lotus.

But she can *move*. She can *breathe*. And most days, she can meet herself where she is. When she does, she remembers to allow space for new insight. Sometimes, Sarah can do full wheel without crushing pain in her low back. Sarah has seven herniated discs in her back, a few of which are in her lumbar spine, and she had been convinced for years that upward facing bow *urdhvadhanurasana* was one of those "pushing yourself to the point of pain" postures for her. That is, until she had a gifted teacher guide her and tell her to think of the opposite of fear as she was about to lift up into the pose. For Sarah, that word is *"courage."* She silently says, *"Courage, courage, courage,"* and every once in a while, it gives her wings.

Yoga and belief bridged the gap for the authors of this book and paved a path to long-term healing for them, and we have seen it do this for others. A key component to allowing these mindfulness practices to be healing is to meet yourself where you are instead of judging yourself. Remember, your body is a good friend, a resource; ask it what it needs. "Meeting yourself where you are" is a dance between complacency and perfectionism, coupled with trusting that you are stronger than you think you are. It's not about finding a perfect balance; it's about being comfortable with the rhythm of your authentic ebb and flow, your surges and drawdowns, learning what your true center is, where you can align with it and bounce back to it after a stressful or challenging time. Learning to find your intelligent edge that fosters growth, versus pushing yourself to further injury, can take a lifetime to master.

Yes, we've been through some very tough times, and so have you. So let's also celebrate the small wins; the daily activities that we *can* do better because of choice based on intuition, agency, and breath; the more compassionate courses we take with ourselves and others; the activities we choose; the food we choose; the decisions we make; and the paths we walk.

Yes, yoga and deep belief in something bigger than herself "saved" Sarah, but it was the breath that softened her. The breath gave her the tangible thing to sustainably anchor to. Breath was a gateway to believing in her own power again, the power to choose her path, the power to heal, and the power to connect. Breath was a vehicle for choice based on mind-body awareness.

Choose one thing you can do. Sarah chose the mat. What's your mat? What moves you from frenetic to calm? What helps nudge you into a "flow" state of mind and being? Where do you heal?

Because as you heal, you create space for others to heal. As you succeed, you give permission for others to succeed. Never stop trying to bring more light, love, and health into your life and into this world. You are worth it. And we need more connection, self-care, belief, and choice in our lives; we need deeper and bigger breaths, and we need to believe in the power of our own intuition, agency, and awareness. We need to embrace humility and humor and presence more than pretense and perfection. We need more love, friendship, and compassion. We need to reflect without ruminating and then move on to be *in* the lives we've crafted for ourselves with the people we love.

You may not think you want to get into yoga and meditation, although both practices offer the nervous system regulation needed to build resilience. Although mindfulness-based practices such as breathwork, meditation, and various forms of yoga are well-studied and validated to make a positive impact on quality of life, vast research also shows that simple, daily physical activity of any kind adds immense value as a self-care practice. Physical activity includes not just the type of fitness we build at the gym, but all types of daily movement both alone and in group settings, getting fresh air, spending time in nature without constantly being tethered to technology, or any other pursuit of a life less stagnant.

The bottom-line up front is this: find a form of movement you enjoy and do it regularly.

Even though Sarah's been an athlete her whole life, she's had seasons when she struggled to incorporate movement into her daily routine. She yo-yoed between pushing herself really hard for any number of weeks or months and then retreating to inactivity for days and weeks at a time. It didn't feel healthy, but she didn't know any other way either. Her weight, mood, and mental acuity hit highs and lows that corresponded with what she was doing physically. It wasn't until she shifted her perception of fitness from "exercise" to "movement" that her mind and body also shifted in a healthier direction in a much more consistent manner.

For example, Sarah had a client who used to be in the Special Forces. After leaving the Army, every time he'd try to "get back in shape," he'd go full tilt, run and lift hard for a few weeks, and then get injured and spend twice as long after that little spurt of frenetic activity doing no exercise at all because he was hurt. During each one of those breaks, he would go longer and longer without activity, and every time he wanted to get back into "working out," it was harder and harder to do so. It never really occurred to him to just ease his way back into things or to still go for a short hike or something on the days he wasn't following a prescribed workout. The hard exercise he was allowing himself did nothing to decrease his stress or downregulate his nervous system. Since cortisol impacts digestion and weight gain (as discussed in a previous chapter), he was actually hampering his fitness efforts. Slow can be strong.

Therefore, when he and Sarah began working together, she encouraged him to *just get moving* again. She told him, "Keep it simple. Don't even worry about running, lifting, or doing anything strenuous. We just want to start by adding movement and fresh air to your daily routine. We'll progress as we go, and that will make this exercise regimen an actual lifestyle versus a sporadic inconsistency." One month in, he felt great. *Three months later, he'd lost 30 pounds and said he felt the best he had in years*. He gradually added in jogging, yoga, and more vigorous hikes to his "just get out and move" goal, and now his longer-term goal to run a Tough Mudder this year seems attainable. *This* is a lifestyle of wellness he can maintain.

Yoga is not the only way to regulate the nervous system or begin to use breath to carve space for making tough calls. Many health practices can make a difference, and a good plan is to try one or two at a time, gradually working them into habits.

A small shift that Sarah found very helpful early on in her healing journey was to think more about "adding in" some "good" things in order to "crowd out" the "bad" things. She began to more often consider things that nourished her and fed her on *all* levels, and as she added in more and more of those things, they crowded out the bad stuff. This concept is applicable with *anything* from food to relationships! In the military, we were taught to reinforce success, not failure. We should keep reinforcing the things that *work*, one little bit at a time, and trust that the compound effect of those small choices end up making big differences in the long run.

We basically have two major coping mechanisms to deal with pain, stress, and anxiety: we either cognitively fuse into our thoughts and get stuck in them as we ruminate on our problems and cannot see or feel anything else or engage with anyone else or we deny, tune out, and ignore. We implement experiential avoidance via lots of creative approaches such as overworking and feeding the chronic busy beast, excessively working out, or using drugs or alcohol. Unfortunately, our problems never go away by ignoring them. So we've got to be *present*. Sometimes being present is downright painful and we don't want to feel that way, but it's part of the healing process. The process can start by choosing to do things that are seemingly simple. Conscious breathing is a simple powerful first step accessible to all of us.

We'll give you some personal examples of things we've "added in" the last few years that we previously thought were silly, or didn't imagine to be that impactful, that we now wish we had learned to do many years ago. We've seen these practices make an impact on our ability to become healthier and healthier after trauma:

- consciously breathing on a daily basis;
- making quality sleep a real priority;
- seeing prayer as a practice, not as an obligation;
- recognizing the value of relationships and ensuring we experience at least one personal connection a day;
- practicing some form of mindfulness almost every day;
- spending time in nature (anything from a few minutes in a local city park to long trips in the wilderness)
- implementing simple self-care practices that are cheap and not time-consuming like body brushing, tongue scraping, and proper skin care;
- eating less processed food and adding in nutrient-dense foods;
- getting massages;
- trying things like acupuncture and chiropractic care; and
- moving every day (not exercise but daily *movement*)—giving ourselves permission, for instance, to take a little walk if we don't have time for a long run. When we consider that trauma lives in the body, we need to *move* our bodies in order to *move through* trauma.

Also, we've made big, scary choices like starting a family of our own, adjusting relationships by letting go of ones we've had for a long time but no longer serve us or the other person, creating better boundaries with family, starting a business, writing a book, testifying to Congress, traveling alone, or playing new sports.

The good news is that you can do these things too. We saw others doing similar things and began to emulate them. Sarah, for instance, moved to a new city and joined an Australian Rules football team to meet new people. As kids, we have teachers and coaches, or in the military we have commanding officers and staff noncommissioned officers as mentors, and then

as adults or when we get out of the military, we often forget their importance. Mentors and peer support matter—we can still have people like that
in our lives!

Every success story includes others. Don't be afraid to ask for help.

Start with one of these things:

- find a fellowship group at your place of worship or a volunteer group in
  your community,
- get a professional mentor or coach (there are many free resources for
  this for veterans),
- connect with a veteran service organization that provides fitness
  groups within which you get the additional benefit of socially connecting in a variety of ways,
- start moving every day, try yoga or other forms of synchronized movement shown to benefit our nervous systems
- drop your soda habit, and
- start with three minutes of breathwork in the morning if you don't
  have twenty.

You don't have to do it ALL, all today. *Choose to start.*

Via these examples, we hope to encourage you to strive to accept the
rhythm of life. No need to achieve a type of balance associated with perfection; rather, keep in mind that some days you'll train harder than others, and sometimes you need to just plain get outside and get moving
regardless of what exactly it is you're doing. You don't always have to be
"working out" for it to "count."

So, find an activity you *enjoy*. Start there. Do it every day.

VETERANS SALUTING THE SUN FOR A CHANGE[2]

** "Sun salutes" or "sun salutations" are a common series of
movements in most "flow" yoga classes*

Sun's fingers reach
over the hills
(pausing first, of course, to inhale the beauty of that recently swollen
    river and admire his own reflection along the way),
through the trees,
and around the pavilion pillars.

Light Breeze, she travels with the Sun,
and reaches, sweeps, dances

over the warriors, too,
as they breathe,
stretch,
and move.

Surely some of them—if not most—are seeing different scenes
    through their mind's eye,
of fields like the ones near them now, but drier,
of hills, but flatter,
harsher,
of wind beating them brittle,
bites more searing from bullets, not bugs,
begging to bring them back,
back to somewhere not *here.*

A fidget ripples through the bunch,
they try to dislodge the begging,
their discomfort visible.

Then we wait . . .
Breathe,
stretch,
move.

A pause.

Again, the ripple.

We wait.

Breathe,
stretch,
move.

Repeat.

Breathe, fellas!

Breathe in,
lift up.

Breathe out,
fold forward.

Ripple.

Repeat.

Breathe in.

Breathe out.

Then
they're there: *Here.*

Now.

Even if for just an instant,
but *Here* they are,
beautiful.

Pain and hope,
siblings in the same body,
as they finish their sun salutes.

NOTES

1. There are many scientific studies that highlight the benefit of breathwork and meditation. Both help the brain reach a state of relaxation where restoration can increase working memory capacity growth. Harvard Medical School. (2014). *Breath meditation: A great way to relieve stress.* Accessed March 20, 2020, Available at https://www.health.harvard.edu/mind-and-mood/breath-meditation-a-great-way-to-relieve-stress

2. This previously unpublished poem was written by Sarah, when she felt especially inspired by a group of veterans at one of her yoga classes in Colorado. Sarah and another Marine veteran, Jarell Jones, started the yoga program at Denver's VFW Post-1, and they were thrilled with the response from the participants. Plummer Taylor, S. (2020). *Veterans saluting the sun for a change.* Accessed July 29, 2020. Available at https://yogaservicecouncil.org/veterans/sun-salutes

If your idea of self-care is eating paleo and running ultra-marathons, we've got news for you—you're missing out.

Self-care goes way beyond the way you feed or train your body: It's about health at multiple levels. At its core, it requires attention to regulating your nervous system—to regularly giving your brain and endocrine system (your body's network of hormone-producing glands) the chance to calm down and return to normal levels.

This type of self-regulation is important for your physical and mental performance whether you're an elite athlete or an everyday person of any age.

Pain Isn't Always Weakness Leaving the Body

As a veteran, you know that the military does a great job attaching metrics to physical fitness. Servicemembers are required to pay attention to their physicality, and intensity is emphasized. These are good things in many ways. After all, you can't see improvement without testing your body's limits.

However, the military often falls short on the topic of balanced wellness. Many veterans leave their time in service physically broken, with muscular imbalances, and they hold fast to the belief that if training is hurting, it's helping. We might even think that only malingerers, failures, and dirtbags take time to care for themselves.

We are not here to suggest that you give up your high-intensity training. But we are here to say that the whole point of intensity should be about using it to increase your performance in a smart and productive way.

Whether your goal is muscle growth or cardiovascular improvement, attaining your specific training objectives will be easier when you lower your blood cortisol levels (the stress hormones your body produces).

You can do this by practicing self-care and something called "mindful movement."

But Isn't Mindful Movement for Hippies?

Mindful movement is as useful for grunts as it is for POGs and as it is for civilians. Here's what career infantry officer Maj. Gen. Thomas Jones, USMC (Ret.), has to say about it:

> For many years as an infantry officer, I worked feverishly to build resiliency in combat Marines. However, and unfortunately, it wasn't until I was a civilian that I learned that I was missing the central, necessary ingredient . . . to crafting resiliency: a thorough understanding of the physiology of stress within the body . . . I learned that mindfulness enabled me to personally address stressors with positive outcomes.

Mindfulness is a form of self-care, and what it really means is that you're paying close attention to your breath and body so you can discover how to care for yourself. For example, if you notice that you have really tight hips, you should work to correct the problem instead of ignoring it. This type of aware-ness is a very calming thing—we can use breath as a vehicle to connect our (sometimes very) disconnected mental and physical selves, and it can let us know how we need to adjust our training or lives to perform more effectively.

When we're busy and stressed, paying attention to the needs of the physi-cal body is one of the first things to go. However, we can benefit tremendously from figuring out when we're not in a rested state and then working to provide our bodies and minds with opportunities to relax.

Why Are Mindfulness and Self-Care So Good for Me?

When we effectively manage stressed-out bodies and minds, our levels of cortisol (a stress hormone) are lowered. Lowering cortisol is helpful because it improves our brain's ability to function and our body's ability to perform.

Alternately, high levels of cortisol encourage your body to seek out and crave simple carbs and store them as fat. Too much cortisol also impairs upper-level cognition in our brains—making it harder to think clearly, experi-ence empathy, and communicate effectively. It can also degrade our physical performance.

Finding ways to lower our stress—even if only for a few moments—has the opposite effect and is incredibly beneficial to us.

So what does a drop in stress hormones feel like? Think about the last time you enjoyed an activity or training—when you took a deep breath in and you just felt that "Ahhh!" feeling—even if you were working hard and running up and down trails. You may find it while running, skiing, doing yoga, getting a deep tissue massage, or even lifting weights. Some people call it a "click," or a "shift."

That moment will look different for everyone, but when you find it, take note.

If I Want to Practice Self-Care, Where Should I Start?

The first and most important step to practicing self-care is to commit to managing your time so you can structure a plan for success.

Next look at how what you're doing on a daily basis makes you feel. Tune into that and take notes for a few days. Do you feel depleted at the end of a day? Energized? Hopeless? Keyed up?

Once you have a read on how you're doing, begin to expand your skills. If you only know one or two tools to make yourself feel better, the good news is that you have lots of room to grow. Continue to do what you already know you like and benefit from, then learn and add in a couple of new options to your wellness program and nutritional choices.

Pay attention to how you're treating your body with food. Consider taking fast food and soda out of the options column for yourself. If you don't want to take them out, then look at adding items that taste amazing and are healthy. Instead of restricting, add in.

If you feel overwhelmed as you think about all the training and wellness options out there, consider plugging into an organization or nonprofit that can teach you helpful skills. As a veteran, if you can imagine a self-care or mindful movement option, a nonprofit probably exists that supplies it.

Self-Care Resources

- Outdoor Odyssey—They provide funded weeklong retreats for wounded, ill, and injured active-duty and veteran warriors, which are designed to craft a definitive plan for the future with the support of a team. They are designed and operated by those who have been there!
- Outward Bound—Operation Iraqi Freedom or Operation Enduring Freedom (OIF/OEF) veterans can enjoy all-expenses paid week-long trips rock climbing, dog sledding, sailing, and more, as they learn the value of compassionate leadership.
- Team RWB Athletic Camps—Learn how to rock climb, practice yoga, or run trails at these camps.
- Sierra Club Military Outdoors—Here, experience power ski, ice climb, whitewater raft, and more alongside fellow veterans in some of America's most stunning backcountry.

SECTION 3

Social Support

8

The Science of Social Health

The last decade of war has affected the relationship between our society and the military. As a nation, we've learned to separate the warrior from the war. But we still have much to learn about how to connect the warrior to the citizen. . . . We can't allow a sense of separation to grow between us.[1]

—Gen. Martin Dempsey, Chairman of the
Joint Chiefs of Staff, 2013

The Department of Defense and the Veterans Administration work tirelessly to provide treatment options for servicemembers with depression and stress injuries. Over the last decade, tremendous strides have been made in regards to availability of and access to care. Within the military community, the entire issue isn't about lack of screening for depressive disorders or in the medical care available to servicemembers suffering from depression. Rather, a huge unspoken part of the problem is getting veterans to *use* treatment services.

One large, post-deployment study of reserve and National Guard soldiers coming home from Iraq revealed dismal mental health numbers. Forty-two percent of soldiers surveyed were flagged as being in need of evaluations and possibly treatment. Only half of that flagged percentage actually went to their evaluations. Of the half who did agree to seek help from therapists, only 30 percent followed the basic program through the full eight sessions.

A major reason that servicemembers avoid treatment is that recommendations to seek it often come from civilian mental health providers. The military is an insular world, and well-intentioned providers are simply not a part of it. As discussed in previous chapters, research has shown that after deployments, separating servicemembers feel incredibly disconnected from civilians.

At no time in Kate's military career was this feeling stronger than right after coming home from Iraq. She served with the Second Military Police Battalion in Fallujah for much of 2005. She felt most days like she was part of something important, surrounded by people for whom she would do anything, and that her work mattered.

The Marines Kate worked with meant more to her than anything in the world, and that feeling was mutual. It was proven in very practical ways in Iraq.

As Military Police, one of the things Kate spent time doing was traveling around the country to meet with Iraqi corrections officials to discuss how things were being done in their prisons. On a trip down to Al Hillah, her group stayed aboard a joint base with soldiers from Mongolia and Poland. As a woman in Iraq, you are stared at frequently no matter where you are, but among the Mongolians, Kate looked like a blonde giant and received a lot of funnier-than-normal looks.

The day after arriving, Kate and her team left the wire to visit the local prison, which happened to be one of the few facilities that held incarcerated women. The women's prison, if one could even call it that, was a single room with a drain in the center of the floor. Women of different ages were being held there, some with their toddlers sleeping next to them on the concrete floor. The translator told Kate that there was nowhere else for the babies to stay and no one else to care for them. Social services weren't coming to help those little ones.

Back on the base, Kate went to sleep, holed up in a disintegrating barracks room with a plywood door. Her fellow Marines were next door; they knew the group only had a few hours to close their eyes before leaving to head back to Fallujah.

Sometime in the dark of night, Kate jerked awake. She didn't know immediately why, but she felt the overwhelming need to be alert. She reached for her service weapon, which was reassuringly nearby, as always. Suddenly, the plywood door was shaking as someone started to pound on it and try to push it open.

The language outside the door was foreign, and their words were slurred with alcohol. The rape risks facing women on overseas bases were no secret, and Kate knew what was happening immediately. She assumed being aggressive would lend better advantage than sitting quietly while they broke the crappy door down. Kate moved toward the door with a

9mm in hand. As she opened it to see two Polish soldiers drunkenly trying to push their way in, the Marines in the hut next door flooded out.

What the "f—" are you doing here at her door?

The soldiers mumbled apologies and left hurriedly in a fit of self-preservation, both disappointed and embarrassed. Kate didn't feel afraid, though she knew their intentions were likely nefarious. She was armed and had her people nearby. She felt lucky to be part of that team.

Kate's experiences in Iraq on convoys and with incoming indirect fire were characterized by excellent timing and good fortune; she came home totally unscathed by either contact or injury. The most she ever saw on the road was a controlled Improvised Explosive Device (IED) detonation. That is a pretty rare thing to be able to say, and for many people she loved, this wasn't the case.

Kate had always been close to her younger brother. He was a Marine Corps Infantry Officer, and when she was near the end of her stint overseas, his was just beginning. Stars aligned when his unit flew in, and Kate had just convoyed down to the Forward Operating Base where they were to arrive. She was able to get to the hangar around the time his unit was landing and be there waiting for him. She still remembers watching him getting off the C-130 with all his gear. He looked like a 10-year-old to her, buried in a rucksack with big, blue eyes peering out from under his Kevlar helmet. She wondered for a moment how his unit had let a kid on the flight.

Kate's heart sank when she saw him, and for the first time since arriving in Iraq, she allowed herself to feel reality. She knew where his guys were headed, and it terrified her. Ramadi was a bad place in 2005; they all knew that.

A month later, Kate was landing safely in North Carolina as an Improvised Explosive Device was changing the world of several Marines and a young Navy corpsman forever. Her brother was in that vehicle.

Thank God, he lived through the experience, but it crushed him that not all the Marines with him did. He was medically evacuated to Ramadi Surgical, then Baghdad, then Germany, and then Maryland. Kate was so grateful for the chance to spend hours by his recovery bedside in Bethesda Naval Hospital—it was better than the alternative funeral at Arlington Cemetery.

For Kate, it was the beginning of a really confusing time. She was home, but home didn't feel reassuringly familiar anymore. Some nights Kate spent in the hospital lounge and many others with family and friends in the D.C. metro area. She would leave the hospital and spend time in the "real world," but it was a world no longer recognizable. Everyone seemed so casual and happy, oblivious to the pain and sorrow facing the young men she had just left in Ward 5. Kate didn't know how to speak to civilians, and her resentment of their complacency seethed under the surface. She was simply angry with no articulable words for why.

Kate got a bit self-destructive that month.

In truth, her struggles connecting with even well-loved friends and family whose lives were untouched by the wars were far from unique. She stopped wanting to speak to anyone who didn't speak her chosen language of alienation and latent anger.

Today, Kate can look back and bemoan her lack of awareness about reintegration, but having tons of coping skills may not have mattered, either. Lots of people had the same issue. Kate was struck reading the story of a professional who was formally trained in combat stress and skillful reintegration. She knew more than anyone how to avoid feelings of disconnect, yet she herself was not immune. A mother and Navy mental health provider, Dr. Heidi Squier Kraft returned from serving with the Marines of al Anbar to return to stateside practice. Of the experience she wrote:

> And so I returned to life as a clinical psychologist in a peacetime hospital. Despite my clinical knowledge that each individual's suffering is real and important, I often found myself staring in disbelief at my patients. I could not fathom the crises that my patients made out of their life events, nor could I empathize with the petty relationship, work, or financial stressors that brought them to tears in my office. Only months before, I had held the hand of a twenty-two-year-old hero who gave his life to save two of his men. I had witnessed courage in the face of injury and pain, loyalty in the face of grief. Everyday psychological problems not only paled in comparison, they struck me as frankly absurd. Despite the personal toll seven months of war had taken, I found myself wishing I worked on a Marine base. At least then I would know what to say to my patients.[2]

The feeling that American civilian culture was just as foreign as any culture in a far-flung land stuck with Kate, but at the time, she would never have voluntarily labeled herself as struggling. Stress injury like this creates numbness and emotional reactivity that get in the way of family bonds and close friendships. For so many veterans, this exacerbates reconnection issues with family and friends after service.[3]

Social support is vital to mental wellness because it lowers stress levels. It is natural and adaptive for humans to seek connection with one another, and interruptions to those close connections are uniquely traumatizing. Loneliness and rejection feel like threats to life and future stability to our nervous systems, and the result is measurable impact on physical health. Strained social relationships only increase the reactivity in a person already struggling with stress injury.

Scientists have studied social support from a variety of angles, looking at the size of networks, whether or not someone has a confidante, partnership status, and the perceived quality of support received. Having a trusted tribe is good for you. Research examples abound. In one study, medical students who were lonely had depressed immune systems. In another, unmarried cancer patients died at greater rates than married peers with the disease. Even elderly dementia patients with more friends stayed sharper longer than their lonelier peers.[4]

Social support is a known contributor to health and longevity, with recent studies indicating that high levels add 7.5 years to the average American life span. Researchers didn't always talk about social support and the vital role it plays in our ability to grow through traumas. In fact, the first study on this phenomenon happened by accident at a medical conference, when a Midwestern college professor met a local physician in a pub.

The researcher's name was Dr. Stuart Wolf, and he spent his time studying the alarming rate at which heart attacks were on the rise in 1950s' America. His new acquaintance listened with interest to his talk of lifestyle-created heart disease and offered him an opportunity that sounded strange. He suggested that Dr. Wolf visit his hometown, a small village in Pennsylvania called Roseto. He had been a physician there his whole life and had never seen the heart attacks Dr. Wolf was describing.

Curious, Dr. Wolf visited and found that the small-town physician had been right—people were simply not dying of heart attacks in Roseto. Dr. Wolf would spend the next three decades studying town citizens to find out why.

Although the Italian immigrants who inhabited the town of Roseto drank wine, cooked with lard, and struggled with obesity, they were remarkably healthy and boasted above-average life spans. Their secret was in their social cohesion. The townspeople lived in nuclear families and interacted with extended family members throughout their lives. They didn't live in idyllic harmony, but they were closely connected to one another. They supported one another emotionally, and there was always a neighbor to help a parent keep an unruly child in line. The community was homogeneous and close, living in extended kinship networks that kept families near one another and allowed the elderly to age in the same home as their grandchildren.

Before future generations moved to the suburbs and increased their work hours, divorce rates, and the stress in their lives, rates of heart disease within this community lay exponentially below national averages, though lifestyle behaviors were far from heart-healthy. The primary difference noted among the first and second generations of study participants was the uniquely warm and cohesive community relationships typical in the small town for first-generation inhabitants.

Dr. Wolfs' thirty-year study highlighted the vital importance of close, nurturing relationships to human health and what came to be known as the "Roseto Effect." Social support can improve anyone's life, but studies have shown that specifically in military settings, high levels of perceived social support independently predict coping with self-efficacy post-deployment.[5]

*   *   *

Not all veterans lose their social support systems upon returning home, though many of us do. It can be tough to stay close to people when we aren't sure that we speak the same language any longer.

Some veterans are blessed with the ability to keep communication lines open even in hard times, and with loved ones they are able to weather the storm alongside. These are the cases that highlight even more powerfully the importance of connection, and Kate will always be grateful that this was her brother's experience.

She was already deployed in Iraq when her brother e-mailed her to share that he was probably going to propose to his girlfriend before he headed over. She was a civilian schoolteacher from Philadelphia whom Kate had yet to meet, and Kate rolled her eyes when he shared his romantic plans. At that time, Kate was surrounded by guys losing their girlfriends to the grind of deployment, and she expected that his schoolteacher would be mailing him the same "dear John" letter after a few months. She told him that she didn't have a problem with the proposal, but cautioned him to buy his beloved a ring made out of cubic zirconia. No sense in buying a diamond he might never get back.

As younger brothers often do, he ignored Kate's advice and bought a beautiful ring.

*   *   *

When her wounded brother arrived in Bethesda, the family didn't know what he might be facing. There was so much damage. On his third surgery, the physicians in the operating room took a vote about whether or not to amputate his leg at the hip; he had infection setting in, and they were worried it could get worse. Two voted to amputate, and three voted to give him a couple of days.

Ward 5 was a dark place some days. Kate and her family were surrounded by morphine drips, pain, injury and struggling families who weren't sure what to make of it all.

Into this world walked her brother's civilian schoolteacher.

She's a civilian—she won't be able to handle this.

She'll fall apart any minute.

She never did.

When her leave ran out at work, she went back to teaching all day long in nearby Virginia, but she made the drive every night to sleep in a chair at his bedside. Kate would find her sitting by her brother's side laughing about some silly thing or another, always keeping him smiling. She never complained and never gave up, and she never confessed fears about marrying a man with so many new health issues.

While Kate fumbled gracelessly in his hospital room, once even dropping a portable DVD player on his gaping wounds, she was all kindness and poise. She kept him looking toward their future on a daily basis—even when he left the hospital and had to spend long days in a reclining chair, even when he needed help with any and all of the most basic tasks.

She helped him through medical retirement and the search for a new career and a civilian identity, and they became parents with that joyous excitement reserved for newbies who don't yet know how much sleep they will soon go without.

She married a Marine with three sisters, all of whom would gladly hide a body for her today—no questions asked.

She has a good memory, though. Every now and again, Kate hears about that cubic zirconia comment.

NOTES

1. A 2015 article in the *Los Angeles Times* highlighted the cultural and geographic schism that currently exists between mainstream civilian society and the military. Less than a half of 1 percent of the U.S. population is in the armed services today, and most servicemembers hail from southern states and families with military service histories. There is truly a divide. Zucchino, D. (2015, May 25). U.S. military and civilians are increasingly divided. *Los Angeles Times*. Accessed January 21, 2020. Available at http://m.military.com/daily-news/2015/05/25/us-military-and-civilians-are-increasingly-divided.html?ESRC=todayinmil.sm

2. Heidi Squier Kraft's excellent book *Rule Number Two* explains the challenge of reintegrating into the civilian world post-service and post-deployment.

3. Stress injury leads to emotional reactivity and a decline in the ability to connect with others, feel compassion, and interact in socially normative ways. This often creates a vicious cycle for veterans coping with trauma; the social support they desperately need to recover is lost in the close relationships damaged by existing symptoms. Cohen, S., Underwood, L., & Gottlieb, B. H. (2000). *Social support measurement and intervention: A guide for health and social scientists.* New York, NY: Oxford University Press; Currier, J. M., Holland, J. M., & Allen, D. (2012). Attachment and mental health symptoms among U.S. Afghanistan and Iraq veterans seeking health care services. *Journal of Traumatic Stress, 25*(6), 633–640.

4. Social cohesion reduces stress levels in humans; we are wired for connection and cooperation. The research basis for such a claim is extensive; well-connected people live longer and suffer less illness and disease than people who are lonely. Specifically looking at mental health conditions like depression

and anxiety, the results are dramatic. Goodwin, J. S., Hunt, W. C., Key, C. R., & Samet, J. M. (1987). The effect of marital status on stage, treatment, and survival of cancer patients. *Journal of the American Medical Association, 258*(21), 3125–3130; Sarason, B. R., Sarason, I. G., & Pierce, G. R. (1990). *Social support: An interactional view.* Hoboken, NJ: John Wiley & Sons; Smith, A. J., Benight, C. C., & Cieslak, R. (2013). Social support and postdeployment coping self-efficacy as predictors of distress among combat veterans. *Military Psychology, 25*(5), 452–461.

5. Support yields trackable physiological, mental, and emotional benefits! Even if relationships are not friction-free, constant interaction with family and friends yields protective health benefits and builds our capacity to grow through trauma. Of course, this is not a guarantee. Partnered and connected people will get ill, but much like a nonsmoker is less likely to develop emphysema, connected individuals are less likely to suffer from a host of health issues. Egolf, B., Lasker, J., Wolf, S., & Potvin, L. (1992). The Roseto effect: A 50-Year comparison of mortality rates. *American Journal of Public Health, 82*(8), 1089–1098.

9

Connecting Post-Service

The need for us to stay connected with one another is incredibly healthy in ways well beyond the feel-good sensation we get from hanging out with friends. As social science and health researchers, we've embraced this conclusion about the importance of social cohesion both through our professional work and in very personal ways. Kate has written about being crippled with shame after a messy divorce and a few years of wildly unhealthy choices. Her inability to share her struggle with others stemmed from a fear of letting anyone see that she was imperfect. Sarah, too, experienced a painful divorce, as well as gender violence and physical trauma that left her with stress injuries, a sense of embarrassment, and mental health struggles she wrestled with—mostly internally—for far too long; for many years, she felt these injuries defined her, and thus they were a barrier to connecting with others because they weren't things she wanted to share.

Barriers to connection exist for all of us. Life has kicked us all in the teeth at least once, and so shame, imperfection, flaws, failures, and more keep us from the very connections we know deep down that we need, connections that directly impact our very day-to-day quality of life.

Social connection impacts the quality of our mental health, our capacity to emotionally regulate, and our physical bodies. We are *wired* to connect in purposeful ways with something bigger than ourselves as well as one another. Thankfully, there are a variety of ways to access those protective factors that can be customized based on personal preferences, interests, and accessibility.

For Sarah, sports have always served as a liaison of sorts, bridging the gap between social groups or during major transitions in her life. While in grade school, being on various sports teams allowed her to make friends among the different "cliques"; in the military, it gave her the opportunity to connect with servicemembers across the branches and to travel to other countries where she also formed friendships. After leaving the military, sports teams have served as a foundation of support and balance, even when she found herself in new cities where she knew no one.

Sarah started playing soccer when she was 4 years old, began swimming competitively at five, and kept adding activities each year. In 2009, she was introduced to one of her now all-time favorite activities: Gaelic football. And in 2011, she discovered something even stranger yet equally fun: Australian Rules football.

These sports have played a pivotal role in Sarah's life because they kept her connected during the times she was at risk of drifting away.

To many outside observers, sports seem like simple diversions, or just another form of fitness and entertainment. But sports, especially team sports, have meant so much more to Sarah than simply serving as a means to get exercise or build confidence. Maintaining participation in familiar sports kept her connected to others in the community, and it connected her to people who broadened her perspective on life.

When Sarah was in the military, both on Active Duty and as a Reservist, she played on the U.S. Military Olympic Women's Soccer Team, or the International Military Sports Council (CISM) team. Even with all the challenges she experienced as a member of that team for many years, it kept Sarah connected in a healthy way. It gave her a social outlet beyond the Marine Corps; it provided camaraderie and companionship beyond the professional realm and with people with diverse experiences. Since leaving Active Duty, other adult-team sports have served the same purpose for her—a healthy social outlet fostering connection and challenging her growth.

Since 2009, every time Sarah has moved, sports have provided an anchor point for her. For instance, when she returned to the Washington, D.C., area after her first big chunk of world travel, although she didn't yet have a job, a permanent home address, or much else in the way of stability, she had a team to turn to for healthy outdoor activity and social interaction. This Gaelic football team was as much a social club as it was a sports one. Then, when she moved to Ohio the following year and found that Columbus didn't have a Gaelic football team, thanks to her then boyfriend (now husband's) investigatory efforts, she discovered another new sport—Australian Rules football—and they instantly had a huge group of kind, new friends in a brand-new town. Beyond the sports, these teammates provided recommendations on care providers, other community resources, and professional networking. The next year, on Thanksgiving Day in Denver, when Sarah was single, alone, and far away from family without holiday plans, her only-a-few-months-old friends from the team invited her to their house for dinner; instead of eating takeout and drinking a bottle of wine alone and passing out on her couch, she spent the afternoon playing touch footy and eating great food with generous people and their families.

If sports aren't your cup of tea, that doesn't exclude you from the ability to connect in a very similar way. We encourage you to find your "football" wherever you go. There are so many teams, clubs, service groups, and social organizations today that there is absolutely no reason not to go out there and get involved and get connected.

We simply cannot weather all of life's storms alone; we're not meant to! We need teammates, mentors, coaches, companions, and leaders in our lives. Even if we do have it all together, so to speak, we still need someone to keep us on track and guide us, to help us continue to grow. Our teachers, teammates, and coaches probably provided that for many of us throughout our childhood. As adults, most of us neglect that need, but we shouldn't! Adults need coaches, mentors, and support systems, too! Perhaps even more so because other than work, what source of mentorship or leadership do most of us have?

But there's a "but," because meaningful team, organization, social, and personal connections require vulnerability, and vulnerability requires relinquishing control, a facade of perfectionism, and often even some underlying shame. Vulnerability is scary. It, too, can be practiced though. Start in small, manageable chunks of vulnerability. You don't necessarily have to share your entire life story from a public stage; maybe just go to a community board meeting for starters or play a couple of games in a city kickball league to get the ball rolling.

So many of us are so terrified of being vulnerable that we never allow ourselves to fully engage—fully *connect*—with others and to be completely excited about how we are living our lives. We keep walls up to keep people out and our excitement down. To what end though? You have "protected" yourself, but you also prevent yourself from experiencing the full realm of emotions that life has to offer.

Sarah admits that it might seem a little silly, but she gets so amped up for all her sports activities even as a grown woman! She gets to spend time with friends, many of whom come from very different backgrounds than her; she gets to travel and compete, connect and work hard, relax and have fun. What might your connector be?

Personal connections can be the cornerstones of your health and well-ness, and they are the required elements of true engagement with life at its fullest, which build resilience. We nourish ourselves in so many ways, not least of which is how we feed our soul by pursuing our passions and plac-ing importance on relationships, through which all of us eventually end up feeling more fulfilled, focused, happy, and excited about nearly everything in life. Regardless of what we eat, or what exercise we do, how we connect is the most important health choice we can ever make.

Section Summary

You're 11 years old, standing in the middle of the school lunchroom with your meal tray. As you gaze over the top of your sandwich, anemic vegetables, and cookie snack pack, you anxiously wonder who will make room for you at their table.

Whether we're 11, 27, or 80 years old, our human bodies read social anxiety like a physical threat. Will you be able to find and keep food? Experience physical safety? Find meaning in work and life? Throughout history, all of these things have been made exponentially more difficult to find without a tribe or group.

Today, we know that being disconnected from others and feeling lonely is extremely dangerous to your health. In fact, it's even more dangerous than smoking.

Stress hormones surge when you're feeling lonely or rejected, and when they're elevated too long, you may begin to have difficulty communicating, displaying empathy, or engaging in high-level thinking. This makes connecting with others even more challenging, and your isolation can easily become self-perpetuating.

The good news is, you can increase your health and performance at work and home by finding or building a tribe.

The strange but true fact is that there's nothing more important to your physical health than community. This is true even if you're an introvert. It's true even if your tribe embraces unhealthy behaviors such as smoking and alcohol abuse, high rates of divorce, and more.

In the military, your tribe is easy to identify. Your tribe may be your branch of service, unit, platoon, or even fireteam. From the first day of training, you and other members of your tribe are working to overcome challenges together. Camaraderie continues as you train, deploy, and socialize together in the coming years.

In *Gates of Fire*, his epic novel about the Spartan 300, Steven Pressfield writes:

> War, and preparation for war, call forth all that is noble and honorable in a man. It unites him with his brothers and binds them in selfless love . . . There in the holy mill of murder the meanest of men may seek and find that part of himself, concealed beneath the corrupt, which shines forth brilliant and virtuous, worthy of honor before the gods.

For many, military service offers the kind of community they've never experienced. In this community, we may find purpose, self-knowledge, identity, and so much more. Challenged by our tribe, we grow stronger, faster, and ideally into better leaders.

However, when we inevitably leave the military, we may find ourselves unmoored—adrift in a sea of isolation and alienation that threatens to sink us into depression, stress, and declining performance at work and home.

In the age of an all-volunteer military, we often hear about the military-civilian divide. It's not just a divide, though—it's a chasm.

If you're a male veteran, only about 12 percent of peers in your age group have served in the military. If you're a woman who has served, that number drops to 3 percent.

When you leave the military, you'll likely struggle to find people who have a deep understanding of your service, experiences, and the unique culture and traditions of military life. Data shows us that alienation—or feeling out of place—is strongly correlated with post-traumatic stress disorder (PTSD) and other stress injuries. Finding or building a tribe is critical to good physical, relational, and mental health.

When you're part of a group and have a deep sense of belonging, a relaxation response takes place in your body and brain. In fact, every system of your body works better when your relaxation response fires. For example, when you're relaxed and eating a salad, your body absorbs 17 percent more iron than when you're stressed and eating a salad. Being part of a community results in a positive cycle. As you begin your search for a tribe, one of the most important things you can do is stay humble. Don't let your veteran status, and all the good things that come with it, become a limiting factor as you build new relationships. Build relationships with veterans and civilians alike.

On the veteran front, give yourself permission to be around people who understand what you've just lived through. A great starting place is any post-9/11 veteran organization—they'll get you connected with veterans who are in a healthy place. Team Red White and Blue's entire mission is to build social community at the local level—to bring people together. Team Rubicon and The Mission Continues can help you discover purpose through service.

Purpose is also key. Ask yourself what your passion, ideal volunteer work, or dream venture looks like, then get to work. You may find your civilian tribe doing volunteer work, as part of a faith group, or while living your purpose-driven life.

Finding your tribe may feel tough at first, but like most things, it gets easier with practice.

SECTION 4

Spiritual Practice

10

The Science of Spiritual Health

Spiritual health is a phrase with quite a broad definition, subject to interpretation by each person exploring their own. We do not intend to promote any one spiritual path in these pages. Rather, the purpose of this chapter is to make a health case for individual exploration rather than to promote any specific dogma or belief system. A belief system and sense of purposeful connection have value. It is interesting that when we look at the research on faith, religious affiliation is the sort of variable that yields both practical and statistical significance, meaning it matters in people's lives as well as in some statistical model. Scientists have found two religion variables that yield the most significance, even when other related or modifying variables are present. If someone is involved in organized religious practices (gathering attendance, small groups, volunteering) and holds their beliefs about faith dearly (high level of subjective religiosity), they are less likely to suffer from a host of health issues.[1]

Non-organized religious practices are individual and are often conflated with the term *spirituality*. Spiritual practices are often derived from the self-disciplining techniques of religious adherents, though today we often hear them spoken about in a secular sense. Meditation, chanting, and breath work practiced by Christian mystics are discussed in broader, more inclusive contexts today, particularly in spiritual traditions that are focused on internal exploration and self-fulfillment. Sometimes they are talked about in even more secular senses with a focus on performance enhancement.

There is tremendous personal utility and some health benefit to personal, non-organized spiritual practices. However, the majority of religion and health science shows maximum benefit for people involved in organized religious communities, which is why this chapter will focus on organized religiosity and the practices associated with it in our discussion of how to build resilience.

Studies overwhelmingly affirm that reporting a high level of satisfaction with spiritual health promotes resilience and well-being. Much like exercise, religion offers true protective effects against heart disease, depression, and even cognitive decline. Religiosity is correlated positively with improved mental and physical well-being and is important for people coping with trauma. How intensely involved a person is in their faith community strengthens the positive impact it can have. Faith impacts human health psychologically, socially, and physically because most religious traditions encourage healthier choices and philanthropic acts. People who identify as religious have lower rates of mental health problems, particularly depression or depressive symptoms.[2]

BEHAVIORAL BENEFITS OF RELIGIOUS INVOLVEMENT—HEALTHY LIVING AND SOCIAL SUPPORT

Behaviorally, belonging to a religious community promotes healthier lifestyles and offers social support. In a secular social contract, support is both given and offered. People of faith believe that it becomes their duty to offer social support when people are in times of great need, even as illness or personal problems prevent them from giving much back. This may explain why studies show that social support from religious communities yields greater health benefits than other types.[3]

Military personnel are more likely to speak about stressful issues with chaplains than clinicians.[4] As a result, religious leaders have a prominent role to play in helping veterans access help and get plugged back into their communities. Studies back up the simple truth that encouraging faith practices also encourages health and happiness.[5] Communities of faith can be profound sources of social support, healing, and hope for veterans returning home and experiencing the stress and possible trauma of transition.

PSYCHOLOGICAL BENEFITS OF RELIGIOUS INVOLVEMENT—HOPE AND POSITIVITY

It isn't just attendance at religious services that offers healing to people. Belief and connection to a belief system does something unique to us when reinforced through personal practice and supported by a community. Whether speaking from a secular or religious position, the question of purposeful connection always comes up when one discusses human mental health and happiness. A well-known researcher in the field of social work spent years immersed in her interviews with people about happiness, vulnerability, and shame. Dr. Brown's work surprised her. She found that faith mattered a great deal to really happy people. "Without exception, spirituality—the belief in connection, a power greater than self, and interconnections grounded in love and compassion emerged as a component of resilience."[6]

Social psychologists discuss human needs as happening in hierarchy, with the need for transcendence being the highest. In this secular sense, transcendence is discussed as the need to help others seek deep meaning and to discover it for oneself.

Seeking transcendence alone or in groups often requires focused and attentive prayer. Devotional time of this nature alters the human brain in a manner different from the mindfulness meditation appropriate for stress management, which is discussed in other chapters as a self-care and mental fitness training method. While meditation activates the parasympathetic nervous system to calm the body's stress response, focused prayer actually calms the threat response while simultaneously stimulating the brain toward feelings of union with others and with a higher power.

Neuroscientist Andrew Newberg at the University of Pennsylvania has worked with respected research teams to show us exactly what happens during attentive prayer of this sort. The posterior parietal lobe that normally orients us in space and time and offers feelings of "self vs. other" deactivates a bit, while the section of the brain that creates feelings of compassion and empathy activates.

These changes to the prefrontal cortex become permanent over time, as the brain acts like a muscle that can be trained. Neurons and synapses get used to connecting during prayer and cause our compassion and sense of loving connection to one another to grow. Intense long-term contemplation appears to permanently change the structure of those parts of the brain that control our moods, give rise to conscious notions of self, and shape our sensory perceptions of the world.

Psychologists know that rumination and intense self-focus are unhealthy for mental wellness. Most faith traditions encourage a philanthropic focus on others' needs, and prayer's impact on the compassion centers of the brain prompts concern and focus beyond one's own walls. Interestingly, studies have shown that religious Americans are more likely to do anything from donating blood to helping a sick neighbor dealing with depression. Among older adults, 70 percent of volunteer work happens in a religious setting. Americans who self-report going to church give four times the amount of money to charity that their secular neighbors do, and they are more likely to do volunteer work with the poor, infirm, and elderly twice over.[7]

In truth, there is a strong scientific case to be made for the importance of spiritual exploration followed by participation or actions taken in accordance with faith. Spiritual health, whatever form it takes, cultivates health and resilience.

NOTES

1. Understanding the way we use the terms religious and spiritual are important when we discuss the importance of faith to health and resilience. In this chapter, we are explicitly talking about the utility of believing, belonging, and participating in an organized faith community. Koenig, H. G. (2008). Concerns about measuring "spirituality" in research. *The Journal of Nervous and Mental Disease*, *196*(5), 349–355.

2. Faith improves a person's health both mentally and physically and has been shown to be tremendously beneficial for individuals coping with stressful or traumatic events. Neuroscientists are discovering that a belief in a higher power and moral code can be physiologically beneficial in a very trackable way. Dein, S., Cook, C. C., Powell, A., & Eagger, S. (2010). Religion, spirituality and mental health. *The Psychiatrist*, *34*(2), 63–64; Koenig, H. G., McCullough, M. E., & Larson, D. B. (2001). *Handbook of religion and health.* Oxford, UK: Oxford University Press; Larimore, W. L., Parker, M., & Crowther, M. (2002). Should clinicians incorporate positive spirituality into their practices? What does the evidence say? *Annals of Behavioral Medicine*, *24*(1), 69–73.

3. Studies on religion and mental health demonstrate that it helps people cope, connect, and make healthier choices. Koenig, H. G. (2008). *Medicine, religion, and health: Where science and spirituality meet.* West Conshohocken, PA: Templeton Press.

4. Active-duty military personnel are often more likely to speak with chaplains than mental health providers. As such, chaplains are an important referral source for servicemembers who need help for stress injuries or mental health problems such as depression. Kopacz, M. S., & Pollitt, M. J. (2015). Delivering chaplaincy services to veterans at increased risk of suicide. *Journal of Health Care Chaplaincy*, *21*(1), 1–13; Nieuwsma, J. A., Rhodes, J. E., Jackson, G. L., Cantrell, W. C., Lane, M. E., Bates, M. J., & Meador, K. G. (2013). Chaplaincy and mental health in the Department of Veterans Affairs and Department of Defense. *Journal of Health Care Chaplaincy*, *19*(1), 3–21.

5. Biofeedback has provided neurologists with fascinating evidence that faith practices optimize our mental and physical health. Haas, P. (2012). *Pharisectomy: How to joyfully remove your inner Pharisee and other religiously transmitted diseases.* Springfield, MO: Influence Resources; Koltko-Rivera, M. E. (2006). Rediscovering the later version of Maslow's hierarchy of needs: Self-transcendence and opportunities for theory, research, and unification. *Review of General Psychology*,

10(4), 302; Moll, R. (2014). *What your body knows about God: How we are designed to connect, serve, and thrive.* Downers Grove: IL: InterVarsity Press; Newberg, A., & d'Aquili, E. G. (2008). *Why God won't go away: Brain science and the biology of belief.* New York, NY: Ballantine Books.

6. Worthy reading for anyone interested in resilience are books by scholar Brené Brown, PhD. She asks important questions about how authentically we connect with others and with God, and she has coined the term "wholeheartedness" to describe people who display high levels of resilience and self-reported quality of life. Brown, B. (2013). *The gifts of imperfection: Let go of who you think you're supposed to be and embrace who you are.* Center City, MN: Hazeldon Publishing.

7. Faith optimizes individual health and creates a ripple effect in larger communities. This shows up in volunteer work; charitable outreach; and reductions in crime, alcohol abuse rates, and substance abuse. There are several outstanding books on the subject of altruism as it relates to religiosity well worth reviewing! Putnam, R. D. (2001). *Bowling alone: The collapse and revival of American community.* New York, NY: Simon and Schuster; Sherman, A. L. (2011). *Kingdom calling: Vocational stewardship for the common good.* Downers Grove, IL: InterVarsity Press; Yancey, P., & Brand, P. (2010). *Fearfully and wonderfully made.* Nashville, TN: Zondervan.

11

Spirituality in Action

Tension is necessary.

If we believe there is *value* in the conflict we all face throughout life, they are not just *bearable*, the struggles will have meaning.

We are *meaning-making* beings after all; meaning gives us a sense of *purpose*, and purpose enables us to weather just about any storm that life sends our way.

This concept shows up in so many aspects of our lives. For instance, the person who happily works the menial job because they know it financially provides for their family in a time of need is able to work that job day in and day out more sustainably than the person who angrily sees no purpose in the job deemed below them. If our hip flexors weren't at least somewhat tight, we'd be limp noodles. If our muscles and bones didn't get pressure from movement and exercise, we'd actually be weaker. If our intellect is never challenged, we'd simply not be as sharp. If our leadership is never tested, our skills would fade.

> Thus, it can be seen that mental health is based on a certain degree of tension, the tension between what one has already achieved and one still ought to accomplish or the gap between what one is and what one should become. Such a tension is inherent in the human being and therefore is indispensable to mental well-being. We should not, then, be hesitant about challenging a man with a potential meaning for him to fulfill. It is only thus that we evoke his will to meaning from its state of latency.

I consider it a dangerous misconception of mental hygiene to assume that what man needs in the first place is equilibrium, or, as it is called in biology, "homeostasis," that is, a tensionless state.

What man actually needs is not a tensionless state but rather the striving and struggling for a worthwhile goal, a freely chosen task.

If architects want to strengthen a decrepit arch, they *increase* the load that is laid upon it, for thereby the parts are joined more firmly together. So if therapists wish to foster their patients' mental health, they should not be afraid to create a sound amount of tension through a reorientation toward the meaning of one's life.[1]

Why do sunsets have such universal appeal?

One reason is because they embody both light and dark. It is a place of transition, one could even argue tension (the light and the dark fighting against one another). A journey from one place to another. We watch in awe and wonder.

And the tension is required to create the beauty.

Et Lux in tenebris lucet—and the light shineth in the darkness.

As humans, we are hardwired for purpose and connection to something bigger than ourselves and to a carving out of and living up to our deepest purpose. Faith is about relationship, and faith is a *practice*—something to be experienced and lived out. We don't just *feel* faith; we can *live* it!

Research on spirituality and health, and the personal stories from many of us, points toward the truism that purpose and connection matter to us. Whether it's Brené Brown asserting that spirituality kept coming up in her research as a requirement for "Whole-Hearted Living,"[2] Duke University's combination of religion and health sciences research indicating the way faith-affiliation and practice impact health, or resilience studies continuing to show the power of connectedness, we cannot ignore the fact that connection with a higher being, belief, or purpose is what we're wired for.

> *It seems that gratitude without practice may be a little like faith without works—it's not alive.*
>
> —Brené Brown, *The Gifts of Imperfection*[3]

WHAT CAN FAITH IN ACTION LOOK LIKE?

• service or volunteer work,

• generosity,

• gratitude,

• surrender,

• acceptance,

- offering compassion and support *to* others as well as receiving help from others, and
- letting go of the illusion of certainty.

When Kate had her son, she was awash in overwhelming feelings of new motherhood. As a baby, he hated to be put down. She didn't know much better and thought she had to constantly hold him. The result was a very tired Kate who didn't have time to cook for herself. It was here that the women of her church saved her. They set up a meal chart and brought healthy meals by each day. These women knew Kate was moving soon, there was no expectation of reciprocity in their giving. They just gave freely to help a struggling new mom because that is what members of the church did for one another all the time. It was their faith in action. Kate knew it made a huge difference for her growing family, but she didn't realize that this giving was likely good for her friends as the givers too.

"Without exception, spirituality—the belief in connection, a power greater than self, and the interconnections grounded in love and compassion—emerged as a component of resilience,"[4] says Brené Brown in regards to her decade plus of research about shame, vulnerability, joy, and the living of a "wholehearted life." Admittedly, allowing a letting go of control or the things we're habitually used to clinging to is difficult because we're creatures who seek comfort in the tried and true. Yet, there's a sense of freedom that arises when we accept the mystery within faith and accept each moment as being exactly what we need at that point in our walk of life. It allows for a release of the weight of having to figure it all out ourselves and welcomes in surprises. It allows life to be a teacher, not just something happening to us. The letting go, surrender, and acceptance make space for things much bigger and brighter than we could ever imagine on our own.

She went out on a limb, had it break off behind her, and discovered she could fly.[5]

Faith is dynamic and diverse. Within faith, we wrestle with doubt. We wrestle with fear. And that doesn't make your faith any less valuable or "real." It requires courage to admit that we don't know what we don't know all the time. This is a place where we can very practically apply acceptance if we are able to acknowledge, name, and be present with the fact that just because we doubt and worry and become scared at times does not mean we are not faithful. All that dark stuff is wrapped up in the light stuff too.

Faith, as ethereal as it often seems, is also very much about the power of our own thoughts and behaviors. When we offer up gratitude, we are practicing faith. Whether through prayer, meditation, other mindfulness practices, or some combo of all of those, the energy of faith we generate in those moments is real. Trust, patience, and acceptance are siblings of faith because patience requires trust, and trust is built on faith. Behaving in an impatient way indicates a mistrust that things will not happen as they should, and you feel compelled to (try to) control them according to your plan even when everything else around you is telling you to slow down, wait, be patient.

Moreover, in no way are we implying that faith *prevents* challenging things from happening; being faith-filled just means you may have a different, more centered, more accepting perspective on things when you do hit a bump in the road. As we open up space for spiritual exploration, we open up a space for things to unfold in ways we could have never imagined on our own. We may no longer feel the need to control everything because we see things evolving as they should.

The key is *practice* We must practice exercising our "spiritual muscle."

Faith—like love—is great to feel, but it becomes transformative and powerful when it is *done*, when it is put into *action.*

Faith—like love—is a verb.

Faith—like love—is enhanced with gratitude.

Faith—like love—is meant to be experienced and shared.

Faith—like love—is limitless.

Faith—like love—exists along a spectrum. Faith includes doubt, fear, and insecurity. Faith becomes richer when we embrace all elements of it.

Faith—like love—can sometimes be the belief in things unseen, intangible, and unimaginable, from feeling the presence of a higher power or purpose to your belief in your ability to do a handstand when you've never done one before in your life, and everything in between.

Within faith, we actually need the dark and the light.

Viktor Frankl says,

> But in robbing the present of its reality there lay a certain danger. It became easy to overlook the opportunities to make something positive of camp life, opportunities which really did exist. Regarding our "provisional existence" as unreal was in itself an important factor in causing the prisoners to lose their hold on life; everything in a way became pointless.
>
> Such people forgot that often it is just such an exceptionally difficult external situation which gives man the opportunity to grow spiritually beyond himself. Varying this, we could say that most men in a concentration camp believed that the real opportunities of life had passed. Yet, in reality, there was an opportunity and a challenge. One could make a victory of those experiences, turning life into an inner triumph, or one could ignore the challenge and simply vegetate, as did a majority of the prisoners.[6]

Those challenging and dark times deserve a bit of celebration in a way. Those are the times where the best opportunities await. Those are the times in which we have the capacity to utilize what's at our disposal while also transcending it. Within every setback lies a seed for success; within every obstacle lies opportunity.

NOTES

1. Here we quote from Viktor Frankl's book, *Man's Search for Meaning*, once again because it so powerfully depicts the protective health factors that faith or deep belief in some purpose beyond ourselves can have. Frankl was a prominent Viennese psychiatrist before World War II, and he is considered the father of logotherapy that asserts that people's deepest desire is to search for meaning and purpose. Frankl, V. E. (2006). *Man's search for meaning*. Boston, MA: Beacon Press.

2. Spirituality, broadly defined, not specific forms of religion, arose repeatedly in her social science research as a key component of what Dr Brown calls "wholehearted living." Wholehearted living is living and loving from your whole heart, from a place of worthiness, engaging with our lives as both strong and vulnerable human beings. Brown, B. (2012). *Daring greatly: How the courage to be vulnerable transforms the way we live, love, parent, and lead*. New York, NY: Avery.

3. Gratitude is now a well-studied and validated actionable practice to express and apply spirituality and faith. Gratitude can be an action in a number of ways: gratitude journaling, expression of thanks to others, expression of gratefulness to a higher power or purpose, generosity offered to others from a place of inner abundance, and much more. Brown, B. (2013). *The gifts of imperfection: Let go of who you think you're supposed to be and embrace who you are*. Center City, MN: Hazelden Publishing.

4. Spirituality, as it positively impacts resilience, is actually quite broadly defined. This is great news because it gives one the freedom to choose a version of it that most powerfully and personally applies to the individual or their family. Brown, B. (2012). *Daring greatly: How the courage to be vulnerable transforms the way we live, love, parent, and lead*. New York, NY: Avery.

5. Often the simplest poem artfully captures a deeper, broader sentiment of trust and faith. Yamada, K. (2017). *She*. New York, NY: Compendium Inc.

6. Opportunity is truly present even in the midst of the most harrowing situations. Frankl, V. E. (2006). *Man's search for meaning*. Boston, MA: Beacon Press.

Throughout history, humans have often weaponized faith. This makes any discussion of the intersection between wellness and spirituality especially tricky because it can be divisive.

However, as Marines, we're always ready to tackle tough things, and as social scientists invested in teaching veterans how to optimize their performance at home and work, we cannot ignore the compelling data surrounding the positive effects of spirituality.

What Does Spiritual Fitness Have to Do with Anything?

There are explicit, direct, trackable ties between resilient trait cultivation and spirituality. These ties include common-sense connections to things such as behavioral health, social support, and philanthropic leanings and the more mysterious connection between positive thoughts and their impact on us at a cellular level.

From Stanford to Duke University to Oxford, some really interesting research is being conducted globally on the ways in which spirituality and religiosity (self-reported connection to organized religion) can improve everything from healing and recovery time to pain tolerance and longevity. The protective effects faith offers when it comes to depression and anxiety conditions are especially significant.

Many scholars and scientists who are not religious do believe that at some level we're wired for spirituality. For example, at the top of Abraham Maslow's hierarchy of needs sits transcendence—or the human need to connect with something bigger and outside of ourselves.

The protective factors offered by spirituality and religiosity are very powerful—even more powerful than many of the behavioral health practices that the military currently invests in financially. Because of this, the topic deserves a closer look in any honest conversation about building resilience.

So What's the Tie-In to Resilience?

The links between spirituality, religiosity, and resilience can be found in three main areas that are significant not only statistically but also practically in terms of health benefits.

1. **Behavioral health.** People who identify as individually spiritual enjoy a number of benefits at the psychological and neurological levels. However, these health benefits are amplified and extended with higher levels of subjective religiosity—in particular when people take their spirituality a step further and practice it with some kind of community.

    For example, binge drinking and promiscuous sex—which are high risk for our bodies—are generally discouraged by major world religions. Religious people across demographics and age exhibit lower rates of smoking, alcohol abuse, drug use, and almost all risk-taking behaviors than their nonreligious peers. They also enjoy lower rates of depression and anxiety, better mental health, and even a slower progression of dementia.

In short, people who gather around an idea of virtue and live it out with community support are less likely to engage in physiologically high-risk behaviors. This tendency toward healthier living results in better long-term health outcomes.

2. **Social support.** People who are very religious tend to be members of a faith community and enjoy strong social ties as a result

Many faiths encourage both the practice of gratitude and giving to others outside of the social contract (which is essentially the idea that if I do something nice for you, you'll do something nice for me). They prompt members to give to people who can't fulfill their end of the social contract. This is the essence of philanthropic giving, which has demonstrated physical, mental, and emotional health benefits.

Of course, you needn't be spiritual to give generously, but religious Americans give significantly more both financially and in terms of volunteer hours than their nonreligious peers.

3. **Positive thought.** Researchers have found an inexplicable link between the practice of prayer and lowered blood cortisol levels and increased high-level cognitive capabilities. Because the brain influences bodily functions such as heart rate, blood pressure, and the immune system, shifting what happens in the brain through spiritual practice can have significant physical impacts.

In fact, in prayer (unlike in meditation) the relationship centers of the brain light up. The parietal lobes light up too. These lobes are on the side of the brain and allow you to experience feelings of empathy. In the Christian tradition, there's a sacred text that speaks to being transformed by the renewal of your mind, and today we're understanding that spiritual practice can actually grow your empathy and increase your ability to connect deeply with others.

Aren't There Downsides to Religion?

It's true that all of the benefits of a beloved social community can also turn negative. If acceptance lowers blood cortisol levels, rejection raises it. So many people have been battered by faith communities around the world. However, although finding an affirming community of faith is a complicated process, it is also important because it reinforces the helpful behaviors and activities listed above.

If you're curious, but don't have a tradition you feel drawn to, commit to doing some research. Maybe take a cultural literacy course on world religions to orient yourself. Then carve out time to ask yourself big questions in a sincere way. Do some research and some learning and look for an affirming faith community that feels like an authentic choice and fit.

The three pillars of a resilient life are social support, self-care, and spirituality. The individual value of these pillars is backed irrefutably by science, and—when practiced together—their benefits increase exponentially.

Big Question Inspiration

- What has "faith" or "spirituality" looked like in my past? What does it mean to me?
- How would I assess my current spiritual health? Do I spend time on it? Do I think about it at all?
- What do I believe?
- Where do I need to go to learn more?
- Who can I reach out to as I figure this out?

SECTION 5

Reckoning with Resilience

12

Resilience Defined

Resilience is the natural, human capacity to navigate life well. It is something every human being has—wisdom, common sense. . . . The key is learning how to utilize innate resilience.[1]

*   *   *

Sarah was at the tail end of her training program when it happened. She was a month away from being commissioned as an Officer of Marines. She had lived an atypical college life to pursue that goal, training hard at 5.00 a.m. in the morning instead of sleeping until noon after a night out with sorority sisters. She studied hard, broke in boots on early morning hikes, and slept in the mud during training exercises with her fellow midshipmen.

They were a small band, bound together by their desire to push themselves and earn their places in the Marine Corps. They were all close, and they had seen one another through breakups, failed exams, and doubts about their readiness to complete Officer Candidates School. They were Sarah's closest friends, people she simultaneously admired and enjoyed.

She never thought it would be one of them.

She laughs wryly and without humor today as she shares what she used to think about sexual assault. In her naive early conception, rape was always a clear-cut act of violence perpetrated by a stranger in some dark alley. If a smart woman took steps to avoid dark alleys, she would be fine. It couldn't ever happen at the hands of a trusted friend and a member of her Marine Corps family.

But it did. Her world could have crumbled that night, but she compartmentalized like a good Marine and pressed forward, ignoring the nagging voice telling her that she was missing something. She reported the assault and tried not to notice the way her command grilled her about the same details over and over and declined to press charges against her attacker. She spoke to a counselor as her command recommended, avoiding medication and working hard to show her professionalism. She tried not to mourn too noticeably when those few sessions were later used to disqualify her from flight school. She tried not to notice the friends who took sides, and she simply moved forward, doing the jobs she was asked to do, being deployed to Iraq twice, and working hard to avoid that nagging voice. The years rolled by, as they do when we don't pay close attention.

It wasn't until she was alone with her thoughts that it got really bad, and Sarah realized she was looking at her service weapon with a wistfulness that scared her. She had a choice to make—give up or do the hard work of processing a rape that felt like a betrayal at every level.

It was tempting to let the depression take hold, but Sarah had never been a quitter. She didn't really know what was next, but she knew she felt better when she moved and paid attention to her breath. So she did lots of that. She carved space for exercise and for sitting quietly afterward, letting her thoughts come as they wanted, no matter how scary they were.

That was her beginning.

* * *

Whether a veteran leaves the active component with nothing but the happiest of memories or with a trauma history doesn't change the fact that reintegrating into the civilian world is challenging. The experience sinks some of us, and some of us meander through it a bit more easily.

The question of *what makes the difference* fascinates the authors, both personally and professionally, probably because we were such cautionary tales for so long after leaving the Marine Corps.

RESILIENCE—THE THEORY

Any good program designed to help veterans leaving the active component needs a theoretical underpinning. Paying attention to both what has worked historically and to cultural competency saves well-meaning professionals from misdirecting resources in attempts to reach military veterans that simply miss the mark. Behavioral change theories apply what we know about human psychology, sociology, physiology, and culture to health programming.

One commonality that behavioral health models share is a focus on the audience as unique, each priority population requiring targeted interventions. The personality of the veteran population is not the same as others, and a program must be modified according to the perceptions and realities of those it is designed to impact. When working to reach veterans, one must be ever mindful of culture and that commonly understood warrior ethos that renders a focus on assets and strength more useful than one focused on susceptibility or recovery.[2]

Resilience has been most frequently defined as positive adaptation despite adversity, and few theories are more appropriate for working with veterans struggling with reintegration than Resiliency Theory. Resilience can be trained and taught and is useful for both military trauma survivors and an average person with absolutely zero trauma history. Frankly, we can all use more of it. The dialogue surrounding resilience is uniquely appealing to veterans. Studying resilience involves identifying the protective personality traits and behaviors that promote growth and looking for practical ways that programming can strengthen and encourage accessing such traits.[3]

Original research on Resiliency Theory came out of the fields of social work and social psychology, but unlike more problem-oriented theories, it came about after inquiry into characteristics demonstrated by survivors of trauma. Researchers began first by asking the question of why some survivors fared better after difficulty than others who experienced the same events.

Dr. Emmy Werner spent three decades studying children labeled "at-risk." In reality, the stories and backgrounds of these children would break anyone's heart. They came to Werner's social workers from abject poverty and abusive homes. Some had parents suffering with mental illness and were basically orphans. Some actually were orphans without relatives or resources to take them in. She studied over seven hundred children to look for common traits in the ones who managed to rise above their "at-risk" status. To Dr. Werner, rising above simply meant becoming an independent and functional adult, avoiding law enforcement involvement, institutionalization for mental health problems, substance abuse, etc.

Her research found that 36 percent of those children were thriving and achieving success in school, professions, and relationships. They self-reported high levels of happiness and quality of life. They all had some similar qualities and personality indicators, and Dr. Werner codified these as resilient traits. Kids who tested as socially responsible, adaptable, tolerant, and achievement-oriented seemed to thrive, especially if they also had excellent communication skills and high self-esteem.[4]

Follow-on studies demonstrated important resilient traits in other countries and populations, with marked similarities existing in thriving survivors. Dr. Michael Rutter's work with at-risk children in Britain highlighted the importance of having a relaxed attitude, demonstrating high self-efficacy, and having good social support in cultivating resilience. Self-efficacy is the belief that you can accomplish something, and it predicts performance as well as the ability to connect with others.

Efficacious people are more likely to engage in preventive behaviors, adhere to desired changes, and view new challenges as eustress rather than distress. Efficacy is built several ways. Mastery experience builds confidence, as past success makes an individual feel like achievement can be repeated. Vicarious experience contributes as well; efficacious people have seen success in action modeled for them. Typically supported people, individuals with high self-efficacy receive verbal persuasion from respected social connections.

Interestingly, a person's emotional state also contributes to efficacy. Stress researchers have empirically proven that fear, stress, and anxiety set off hormonal chain reactions in the body that elevate blood cortisol and adrenaline. This response limits upper-level cognition, impairs physiology, and reduces feelings of efficacy. A person with high self-efficacy typically knows how to manage their stress. Numerous studies validate self-efficacy as a tool to promote positive health behaviors, and cultivating efficacy has been found to build traits that define resilience.

Researchers repeatedly found in numbers both practically and statistically significant that the ability to self-correct, demonstrate confidence, and exude sociability helped individuals thrive despite dire circumstances and trauma histories. By 1995, researchers had clearly demonstrated a case for the existence of key identifiable traits that made a person resilient. The question moving forward became not whether resilience was real, but whether it could be cultivated.

Put simply, people can train themselves to be resilient for those times when hardship comes unexpectedly. Controlled pressure followed by specific exercises to de-escalate the body's reaction creates the ability to handle more pressure next time. Cultivation is core to the theory's concept; the resiliency model was developed to highlight the process whereby an individual moves through stages of biopsychospiritual (holistic, whole-person) homeostasis. Simple studies have consistently highlighted the model's central premise—that disruption followed by time and self-care aimed at reintegration actually cultivates resilient traits.

Researchers interested in psychological and social determinants of health picked up the concept of resilience, and they have gradually extended its use from the domain of mental health to health in general. Early work on resilience was concerned with the individual, but more recently, researchers have become interested in resilience as a feature of whole communities. Resilient traits can be taught, but this does not happen in a vacuum. Cultural analysis to ensure applicability is vital.

Such cultural consideration defines modern Resiliency Theory; this third wave builds upon existing ecological theory work in public health to consider the multiple layers that impact us as individuals. Ecological theories explain the way that the push and pull of one's environment yields tremendous influence on choices and behaviors. Third-wave Resiliency Theory works to apply questions of environment and culture to any study of individual resilient traits, with the goal being more effective cultivation of those traits by focusing on building them within supportive communities invested in doing the same. This wave is influenced by postmodern, multidisciplinary efforts to identify motivational forces in individuals, groups, and larger communities while simultaneously analyzing context and group experience.

That sounds complicated, but it really just means that the theory is about looking to maximize assets people already have within them in every space they exist, socially interact, and work.

Resiliency Theory as it applies to health behavior change is a powerful paradigm from which to approach research and programming, primarily because it promotes a model of agency and client control. Research has shown that, indeed, much of what seems to promote positive adaptation despite adversity does originate outside of the individual—in the family, the community, the society, the culture, and the environment. A confrontation with adversity can lead to a new level of growth, indicating that resilience is something innate that needs only to be properly awakened.

THE RESILIENT VETERAN

Trying to help military veterans using this theory involves asking them to get involved in their own healing process. It actively discourages victim-identities and speaks to warrior culture much differently than the highly stigmatized clinical intervention model does. Well-known theorist Dr. Richardson wrote of this difference, "The health education and prevention professions are in the midst of a philosophical revolution attempting to build upon negative risk reduction programs, which are driven by the medical model, to competency models."[5]

Applying Resiliency Theory to the military has yielded positive results to date. Post-service, some individuals are more psychologically resilient when faced with reintegration stresses, and we can help train everyone to that standard. For those who struggle with resilience the way we did, increasing understanding of resilience within given communities and populations may help target programming that offers an alternative to the lonely six-pack of beer.

For example, one 2010 pilot study of returning National Guard soldiers completing their deployment to Iraq demonstrated that high levels of resilient characteristics fully mediated the likelihood of self-reported depressive symptoms. If soldiers were categorized as having resilient traits, they did not also report mental health issues. Another study found the same protective effects offered by resilient adaptability in 2013. This Canadian study assessed the criterion validity of a model of psychological resilience composed of various intrapersonal and interpersonal variables for predicting mental health among Canadian Forces (CF) members returning from overseas deployment. Participants included 1,584 male CF members who were deployed in support of the mission in Afghanistan between 2008 and 2010. The results demonstrated the importance of resilient traits in predicting better mental health in Canadian veterans and emphasized the protective nature of conscientiousness, emotional stability, and positive social interactions. The more prominent traits indicating the resilience that a soldier held, the better their mental health after returning from combat.[6]

HELPING VETERANS EXPERIENCE REINTEGRATION CHARACTERIZED BY RESILIENCE

The process of psychological reintegration is the ability to learn new skills from the disruptive experience and to put life's perspective back in a way that will increase abilities to negotiate life events. Serving in the military (whether one went to war or remained in garrison) is a significant disruption to life in an era where so few Americans do so. Military personnel are a minority, and during the return to civilian life, they are faced with disruptive stressors socially, professionally, mentally, and emotionally.

To optimally reach veterans struggling with transition requires reaching out to teach resilience well before that transition begins. There is value in learning to manage stress, hardship, and challenge, and buttressing specific areas of our lives can do that. The challenge for health professionals looking to stem the tide of service suicides and improve quality of life for veterans lies in shifting the paradigm away from a focus on problems and toward theories and methods of resiliency cultivation, preparation, and self-care practices.

While it is tremendously exciting that we are starting to see the value of such piecemeal programs to treat people already struggling, our hope is that we can take another step to insert protective trait training into the active duty world. We can make things better for those who come after us with some savvy programs based on good evaluation evidence.[7]

Both cultural analysis and examination of ecologically focused Resiliency Theory suggest that the ways health promoters bring programs to veterans must emphasize assets and agency. Three decades of evidence provides us with a roadmap to success—the best method for building resilience is to learn and regularly employ techniques to improve social support, self-care, and spirituality.

* * *

Her journey to health and wholeness wasn't a quick one, nor was it handed to her in a prescription pill, but Sarah worked her way into resilience and healing. She received regular counseling, became a yoga teacher and holistic nutrition nerd, and started volunteering a whole lot more. Today she gives speeches about sexual assault and healing trauma, focusing heavily on the role of mindfulness-based resilience-building practices and agentic, holistic health in recovery. She teaches yoga to other veterans today, always making her classes free and accessible for those who might find the mat to be the useful alternative that she did. Shifting her wistful gaze away from the pistol required choice. Replacing unhealthy behaviors with healthier ones involved many changes, and choosing to work and spend time with a trusted tribe of affirming people who valued the same things she did gave her a chance to move forward.

If you ask her, she will tell you that she'd change none of it.

NOTES

1. Resilience has been studied in many different populations, but common personality traits are typically identified in members of each community who demonstrate the quality. Because the traits can be identified, they can be trained and cultivated. Resilience can be taught. Heavy Runner, I., & Marshall, K. (2003). Miracle survivors: Promoting resilience in Indian students. *Tribal College Journal, 14*(4), 14–18.

2. Behavioral change theories help guide our understanding of how to conduct outreach in any population, and choosing one to underpin a program should be done with culture in mind. Hayden, J. (2009). *Introduction to health behavior theory.* Boston, MA: Jones and Bartlett Publishers; Malmin, M. M. (2013). Warrior culture, spirituality, and prayer. *Journal of Religion and Health, 52*(3), 740–758.

3. Post-traumatic growth is an oft-discussed concept that retains a focus on post-incident care and adaptation. It is useful when thinking about veterans working to recover from something traumatic, but it lends itself less to the general,

preventive focus as well. Garcia, B., & Petrovich, A. (2011). *Strengthening the DSM: Incorporating resilience and cultural competence.* New York, NY: Springer; Richardson, G. (2002). The metatheory of resilience and resiliency. *Journal of Clinical Psychology, 58*(3), 307–321.

4. Resiliency has been extensively studied, and key traits make a person more resilient. Most of these traits are related to one's ability to demonstrate self-awareness, adapt, and communicate across difference; Bernard, B. (1997). *Turning it all around for youth: From risk to resilience.* Launceston, Tasmania: Resiliency Associates and Global Learning Communities.

Garmenzy, N. (1991). Resiliency and vulnerability to adverse developmental outcomes associated with poverty. *American Behavioral Scientist, 34,* 416–430; Rutter, M. (1985). Resilience in the face of adversity: Protective factors and resistance to psychiatric disorder. *British Journal of Psychiatry, 147,* 598–611; Werner, E., & Smith, R. (1982). *Vulnerable but invincible: A longitudinal study of children and youth.* Ithaca, NY: McGraw Hill.

5. Noted psychologists and psychiatrists have suggested that competency and resiliency characteristics are strengths that are more protective than risk reduction efforts when it comes to depression. Tested specifically for validity in military communities, protective effects against depression most often emphasize adaptability; Fletcher, D., & Sarkar, M. (2013). Psychological resilience: A review and critique of definitions, concepts, and theory. *European Psychologist, 18*(1), 12–23.

Foran, H. M., Adler, A. B., McGurk, D., & Bliese, P. D. (2012). Soldiers' perceptions of resilience training and postdeployment adjustment: Validation of a measure of resilience training content and training process. *Psychological Services, 9*(4), 390–403; Whiting, L., Kendall, S., & Wills, W. (2012). An asset-based approach: An alternative health promotion strategy. *Community Practitioner, 85*(1), 25–37.

6. Studies have shown that military personnel in possession of known resilient traits rarely suffer from problems after deployment. Lee, J. H., Nam, S. K., Kim, A., Kim, B., Lee, M. Y., & Lee, S. M. (2013). Resilience: A meta-analytic approach. *Journal of Counseling & Development, 91*(3), 269–279; Pietrzak, R. H., Johnson, D. C., Goldstein, M. B., Malley, J. C., & Southwick, S. M. (2009). Psychological resilience and postdeployment social support protect against traumatic stress and depressive symptoms in soldiers returning from Operations Enduring Freedom and Iraqi Freedom. *Depression and Anxiety, 26*(8), 745–751.

7. Empirically validating programs designed to build resilience is an exciting and emerging effort for behavioral health professionals. Lehavot, K., Simpson, T. L., Der-Martirosian, C., Shipherd, J. C., & Washington, D. L. (2013). The role of military social support in understanding the relationship between PTSD, physical health, and healthcare utilization in women veterans. *Journal of Traumatic Stress, 34,* 111–117; Libby, D., Corey, E., & Desai, R. (2012). Complementary and alternative medicine in VA specialized PTSD treatment programs. *Psychiatric Services, 63*(11), 1134–1136.

13

The Health Benefits of Resilient Trait Cultivation

By now, we all agree that there is a problem with the way veterans are transitioning home to civilian life and that this results in some serious public health issues. The question becomes at this point, *how do we make a difference?* Keeping mental health services cutting edge and readily accessible is an important part of the picture, though for reasons discussed in this book's introduction, it cannot be the only answer. Addressing wellness in the military requires a multipronged approach and a holistic focus on individuals in community context. First, we need to focus on savvy programs for veterans who have already served, particularly the younger veterans of Iraq and Afghanistan who are more likely to be walking around with symptoms of undiagnosed depression.[1] Second, we need to develop a prevention focus and do more to make transition smoother for personnel currently on active duty and for those who will serve in the future. Transition education should be more than a one-week class on the way out of active duty, and a focus on resiliency training in the active component can smooth the rougher spots.[2]

If resilience can be cultivated, trained, and taught, we can test for it. We can craft programming that is developed specifically for female veterans, for veterans going back to school, or for veterans with families. We can deliver such interventions with the benefit of careful, focused program evaluation data behind them—making sure that what we are offering is useful, culturally appropriate, specialized, and evidence based. At present, much of the well-intentioned programming being offered lacks real evaluation metrics.

VETERANS LEADING VETERANS

When working with both active duty and veterans, peer leadership is incredibly useful. Warrior subculture creates a powerful mandate for peer-to-peer outreach. Any message aimed at promoting wellness must come from members of the community in order to be deemed credible. Recall that a major sentiment expressed by separating servicemembers is a feeling of disconnect from civilians, especially after a combat deployment.

In the military community, the best program implementation cases are found within participatory research frameworks. Because warrior cultures have their own temperaments, they are typically exclusive and mistrustful of outsiders with different life experiences.

Programs have a chance to work best when veterans or active duty personnel have a hand in planning and implementing them. The 2010 case study highlighted in section one is a terrific example, sharing one Michigan pilot program's experience with "buddy-to-buddy" peer support programs. What made the program uniquely successful wasn't the content; it was the delivery channel chosen. The team of Michigan researchers keenly understood the need for audience-centered communication, and they partnered with unit leadership to institute a program that was completely peer-led. This decision came out of the qualitative research they conducted in the unit prior to thinking about a program. Interviewees said things like, "if you haven't been there, you don't get it" and "other veterans can be trusted." The research team considered concepts of warrior culture and sought to design a program that spoke the correct language, using an understanding of social norms to change the culture of treatment avoidance.[3]

Another reason the success of the program is so noteworthy is that it worked with reserve personnel after deployment. National Guard soldiers, like all reservists, often face stresses additional to those faced by active duty troops. Reservists don't serve within the supportive community of a full-time active duty military component and may lack support services in civilian community settings. Particularly because post-traumatic stress (PTS) symptoms are very likely to be misread as behavioral deviance, stigma may be even more difficult to overcome in community settings removed from the active duty military component.

PROGRAMMING IN COMMUNITIES

There have been exciting successes as motivated nonprofits, academic research teams, and service providers of every stripe have made efforts to help veterans navigate their life post-service and post-war. Too many organizations to name have established nonprofits and worked to provide therapeutic services for military veterans. From animal therapy opportunities to outward-bound adventures, kind-hearted servant leaders have stepped forward to create programs and bridge gaps. These groups offer a hand, a new experience, and attempt to save and improve lives. The Wounded Warrior Project® funds many of these as partner nonprofits and has been instrumental in getting resources out to lesser-known groups.

In particular, organizations created by and geared particularly toward younger veterans of the Iraq and Afghanistan conflict era have brought important opportunities at the community level. They all focus uniquely on empowerment narratives, asking veterans to get engaged as they participate in services and programs, encouraging them to give back, get off the sofa, and plug in to their local community. *The Mission Continues*, *Team Rubicon*, and *Team RWB* are prime examples of groups that work to give veterans a new social community centered around a common purpose. The Bush Institute's Warrior Wellness Alliance is bringing these organizations together to cement best practices and evaluation plans; a network is being created with the potential to dramatically improve the nonprofit space's efficacy.

A PREVENTION FOCUS—TRAINING THE ACTIVE DUTY COMPONENT

Veterans who have also acquired skill sets in the civilian world lend a trusted hand to the process of improving mental health and transition preparation for military personnel before they leave active service. It is incredibly important that in addition to helping veterans currently struggling, we work to prevent those struggles for current servicemembers.

It is important to create programs aimed at post-service quality of life improvement and healing, but the biggest impacts can be made from a prevention angle. The reason for this is that stigma isn't going away, and we can reach more personnel while they are still serving than after they leave. Implementing in participatory fashion in the training environment, rather than in treatment settings, works ideally for veterans who often reject patient identities. That approach works around a major barrier to care for mental health in this population. To combat suicide rates and promote military and veteran mental health, a new approach is required, one that embraces peer education and speaks to the participatory, hard-working ethos of military culture. Resiliency Theory–based programming has potential to meet these needs and may provide a blueprint for success in working with this population.

Creating a climate of peer-led training at both the unit and individual levels will reduce overall stigma against self-care practices because everyone participates, the program is led by trusted informants, and no one has to take on a patient role to participate. To train is to actively participate, and this is a wellness concept with which servicemembers are already familiar. Framing mindfulness training as a way to "bulletproof your brain" renders palatable a training opportunity designed to create more effective warriors with mental endurance; framing this as promotion of combat fitness, resilience, and mental endurance renders it accessible to the military population.

We have to speak the language of warriors when we talk about resiliency cultivation. By establishing mental fitness as another component of optimal combat readiness, we establish resiliency training as a crucial component of mission preparedness and remove the stigma of such practices for post-deployment troops who may be struggling with stress illnesses of varying degrees. The message can become directive; just as Marines and soldiers learn mission essential skills and train their bodies for arduous combat, we must adopt practices designed to train and promote health in the mind, body, and spirit in a holistic sense.

Researchers from all over the country are working to revamp stress management in the military with an eye toward turning management of reactivity into a performance enhancer for the active duty component.[4] Their argument is a sound one. Interestingly, high stress reactivity, naturally occurring adaptation though it may be, hinders the ability of servicemembers to perform complex missions and interact with foreign nationals. The modern battlefield involves interaction with civilians and allies as a matter of course.

Becoming overly reactive as a response to a challenging environment hinders that mission. For example, research has shown that soldiers who screened positively for mental health problems were three times more likely to report having engaged in unethical behavior while being deployed. Behaviors ran the gamut from unnecessary property damage to noncombatant injury or harm, all diametrically opposed to the United States' mission of winning hearts and minds. These issues leave behind moral injuries with which servicemembers may struggle well into their futures.

Again, let us insert our key caveat here. Stress injury is real. When our body's stress response fires at the fight-or-flight intensity level for too long, our nervous systems are going to need help and professional treatment to get back into a regulated state. When we see signs of hypervigilance and reactivity in ourselves or one another, we need to encourage professional assistance and also emphasize that stress injury is a recoverable wound, not a permanent disorder. Trauma, combat, and unchecked chronic stress can create this injury. We need to know the signs and be supportive about seeking helpful services. We need to avoid telling one another to *suck it up.* Just like running another race on a stress fracture is a dumb idea, telling ourselves to push through a stress injury or a case of depression only makes things worse. Help is there for a reason—to get us back into our desired peak-performing state as soon as possible.

However, the stress the veterans face while transitioning to the civilian world does not have to reach traumatic levels and become injurious. Psychologists have done some really exciting studies on mindset interventions meant to help people insert larger context and meaning into their stressors and situate them against a larger mission or set of goals. What they find is that by reminding people of the *why* behind their struggle, they can actually alter the stress hormones released to help create a challenge response or a tend-and-befriend response. These are very different from the intense reactions that can cause injury. These useful forms of performance-enhancing stress make us resilient, effective, and able to handle the mountain in front of us.[5]

DESIGNING PROGRAMS WITH SOLID FOUNDATIONS

Rigorous evaluation of existing outreach efforts provides the foundation upon which savvy programmers must build. Our best chance for making a difference in the training environment before a servicemember faces transition stress involves designing programs from a baseline of proven success. The programs should be tailored for audience appropriateness. Cultural competency means not only trying to understand the veteran experience but also learning the most effective ways to communicate with different subsets of the veteran and military populations.

Health promotion professionals working to prevent and treat mental health problems such as depression and stress illness must understand the confluence of warrior culture and mental health issues in the veteran community. There is ample evidence to support the development of a culturally informed resilience training protocol. Such protocol involves teaching self-care (nervous system regulation), building social support, and introducing the importance of purposeful and contemplative practices. We hope this book serves as a spark for conversation. We hope it renders more complex the question of how to change military and veteran suicide rates. And finally, we hope it assists people looking to live happy, healthy, and productive lives during and after service.

NOTES

1. Kate's research on depression rates in military veterans has shown that the most likely group of veterans to self-report symptoms that indicate undiagnosed depression of mild, moderate, or major severity is the most recent cohort of servicemembers from the Iraq and Afghanistan conflict era. These veterans are more likely to be newly transitioning and are less likely to have successfully navigated access to care issues with the DOD or Department of Veterans Affairs (VA). They also combat strong stigma against mental health care-seeking. In a sample of over fifty-four thousand veterans, only 2.2 percent agreed or strongly agreed that mental health treatment was useful. 97.8 percent held unfavorable opinions about getting clinical help for mental health struggles. Thomas, K. H., Turner, L. W., Kaufman, E., Paschal, A., Knowlden, A. P., Birch, D. A., & Leeper, J. (2015). Predictors of depression diagnoses and symptoms in veterans: Results from a national survey. *Military Behavioral Health*, *3*(4), 255–265; Thomas, K. H., Albright, D., Shields, M., Kaufman, E., Michaud, C., Plummer Taylor, S., & Hamner, K. (2016). Predictors of depression diagnoses and symptoms in United States female veterans: Results from a national survey and implications for programming. *Journal of Military and Veterans' Health*, *24*(3), 6–17.

2. Common transition training for the active component includes a one-week class that all servicemembers complete as they end their time in service. Military personnel receive a great deal of information in firehouse fashion during these transition assistance classes. Opinions on program utility in veteran service spaces are typical in that they do not offer a true bridge between the worlds.

3. Because of military culture insularity, programs that seek to collaborate, bridge gaps, and use peer leadership meet with real success. As has been demonstrated successfully in recovery communities, peer mentoring and leadership provides the interaction, camaraderie, and instructor the credibility required to sell an intervention to potentially recalcitrant participants in very specific, insular, or marginalized communities. Greden, J. F., Valenstein, M., Spinner, J., Blow, A., Gorman, L. A., Dalack, G. W., & Kees, M. (2010). Buddy-to-buddy, a citizen soldier peer support program to counteract stigma, PTSD, depression, and suicide. *Annals of the New York Academy of Sciences*, *1208*, 90–97; Gutierrez, P. M., Brenner, L. A., Rings, J. A., Devore, M. D., Kelly, P. J., Staves, P. J., & Kaplan, M. S. (2013). A qualitative description of female veterans' deployment-related experiences and potential suicide risk factors. *Journal of Clinical Psychology*, *69*(9), 923–935; Held, P., & Owens, G. P. (2013). Stigmas and attitudes toward seeking mental health treatment in a sample of veterans and active duty service members. *Traumatology*, *19*(2), 136–145.

4. Studies of Marines in the fleet during pre-deployment work-ups have looked specifically at the question of whether training can prevent problems after returning home. Results have been positive, and in select studies, statistically significant in the studied population, they demonstrated that adherence to intervention protocol for 15 minutes each day exponentially improved working memory capacity. Working memory capacity contributes to emotional regulation as well as upper-level cognitive functioning. Such findings indicate an affirmative answer to the specific question of whether mindfulness training can promote stress

resilience in a very specific population, at a very critical juncture. Jha, A. P., Stanley, E. A., Kiyonaga, A., Wong, L., & Gelfand, L. (2010). Examining the protective effects of mindfulness training on working memory capacity and affective experience. *Emotion, 10*(1), 54–64; Teng, E., Hiatt, E., Mcclair, V., Kunik, M., Stanley, M., & Frueh, B. (2013). Efficacy of posttraumatic stress disorder treatment for comorbid panic disorder: A critical review and future directions for treatment research. *Clinical Psychology: Science and Practice, 20*(3), 268–284; Thomas, K. H., & Albright, D. L. (Eds.). (2018). *Bulletproofing the psyche: Preventing mental health problems in our military and veterans.* Santa Barbara, CA: ABC-CLIO/Praeger.

5. Stress doesn't have to tear people down. Hardship and trauma can be the fires that hone focus and performance. It is all about mindset and mental fitness training. McGonigal, K. (2015). *The upside of stress: Why stress is good for you, and how to get good at it.* New York, NY: Avery Books.

Young veterans often ask us why they should care about resilience. It's a fair question. At this point, the term is almost meaningless—an overused buzzword. American military culture in particular has packaged "resilience" into a PowerPoint training requirement. It seems like an add-on. An annoyance.

It's unfortunate because resilience practices are key to maximizing performance. And when you're performing optimally, your family, your team, and the other people around you benefit significantly. We're better off in every area of our lives—personally and professionally—when we practice resilience trait cultivation.

The three pillars of a resilient life are social support, self-care, and spirituality. The individual value of these pillars is backed irrefutably by science, and—when practiced together—their benefits increase exponentially.

We promise not to spend the next few paragraphs trying to convince you to drink green smoothies and sit on a therapist's couch. There's a lot more to wellness than that. Instead, we'll examine some simple tactics you can start using today to build a better life.

1. **Self-care: Calm your body and mind**. Start here by choosing just one or two healthy practices you can incorporate as daily habits, then track how they benefit your life. Don't worry about trying to change everything at once.

    By practicing effective self-care to calm your body and mind, you can become less reactive to external stressors. When you're less reactive, you're more capable of engaging in positive social interactions. Better social interactions result in increased social support. Improved social support increases your physical and emotional health. There's a ripple effect here that's really exciting.

    Self-care can be as simple as cooking at home or going back to the gym. What you're looking for is something that makes you feel relaxed. You might be working hard, but you're going to feel your sympathetic nervous system (body and mind) calm down. Some people call it a click. An exhale. A downshift. When you feel it, you'll know you found your thing.

    Think of your sympathetic nervous system like a dashboard: It's where your perception, speech, and moving about in the world happens. It's where you live when you're alert. Our goal through self-care is to pump the brakes and calm down this side of our nervous system.

    When our brains shift to rest, our bodies and minds are refreshed, and we're more capable of controlling our emotions, focusing, and engaging in high-level thinking. You can reach this rested state by sleeping, but you don't have to be sleeping to be in this zone. You may also get there by swimming, snowboarding, gardening, praying, meditating, or hitting flow in some other activity you enjoy. Most of us—particularly those of us with stress injuries—are sadly lacking in this rested state.

As you begin incorporating daily self-care practices into your life, track your progress. Take note of how you feel two weeks in. Do you feel better? More focused? Do you sleep better at night? Are you feeling less pain?

Remember that self-care will differ for every person. For example, if meditation isn't for you and you keep trying it, it can actually increase your stress. You may not be a meditator—you may be a trail runner. It's about trial and error. Don't be surprised if what works for you changes over the years. The most important thing is to maintain your willingness to practice and to understand that it may take time to discover what works best for you.

2. **Social support: Surround yourself with good people**. The first and most important step in building resilience is making the hard choice to surround yourself with great people. If you don't have them around you, you can't get started. You won't start or keep growing.

    This seems like an obvious step, but it's a real challenge for some. It was for us.

    The truth is, you've got a battle ahead and you're most likely to succeed if you have like-minded people to walk with you as you make some changes. I'm not saying you have to hang out with people who look, think, and talk like you, but you do have to spend time with people who are supportive and interested in their own growth and development.

    Take a moment to honestly evaluate the influence of the people in your life. Is their influence negative and destructive or positive? If you don't have great people around you right now, that's OK. It means you have plenty of room to grow.

    You may need to make some serious life changes to find a more positive tribe. You may also need to put yourself in some uncomfortable situations to meet new people. Perhaps you'll find your new group while volunteering, on a sports team, or as part of a faith community.

    If you're not in a great place right now, or you don't have many skills when it comes to connecting with other people, you might be feeling shame or a lack of confidence. Do some outreach anyway. Be willing to risk sharing things that feel deeply personal. You'll be surprised at how supportive people can be when you open up.

    Think about this intense challenge in terms of improving yourself for the people you love.

3. **Spirituality: Find your meaning.** Finally, there's a clear correlation between physical, mental, and emotional resilience and a sense of

meaning in our lives. We all need a connection to someone higher—with God, or a sense of personal purpose. Whether you approach this aspect of resilience from a secular perspective (think Maslow's hierarchy with transcendence at the top) or with a theological view, give yourself some time to ask questions about the source of purpose and meaning in your life.

To plug into a community that supports you as you explore this aspect of resilience, consider getting involved with your church, synagogue, or specific faith group; volunteering; giving generously; or taking time to study a faith practice you've been curious about.

Afterword: A New Approach to Combat Trauma: Healing Veterans and Military Members with Body-Centered and Alternative Treatments

Kate Hendricks Thomas, Pam Pence,
John S. Huang, and Justin T. McDaniel

INTRODUCTION

The cost of war is always greater than originally anticipated, a truth attested by post-9/11 veterans facing mental health issues. However, training to "bulletproof the mind" can keep servicemembers' missions effective in greater numbers, prevent some stress injuries, and treat them if they do occur (Thomas & Plummer Taylor, 2015). In this book, the authors have highlighted the crucial roles of community organizations and individual resiliency practices in preventing military suicide. To that conversation, we intend to add some "tools to the toolkit." We will be exploring the specifics of complementary techniques that offer dual benefits—to treat mental health conditions following military service as well as to prevent poor outcomes before they occur. These therapies, often referred to as "complementary integrative health practices" or "complementary and alternative medicine," are nontraditional modalities that are not mainstream pharmacological or physical treatments (conventional Western medicine) for the treatment of disease or suppression of symptoms. The most common term now used federally is Complementary and Integrative Healthcare (CIH), and it has become common parlance as major changes within the military and the Department of Veterans Affairs (VA) have shifted both the promotion of health and treatment for combat trauma. In addition to evidence-based treatments that have emerged combining psychotherapy and medication, health-care providers have recognized the value of additional approaches to treatment that generally fall under the concept of CIH. These treatment modalities vary measurably and include acupuncture, yoga, health coaching, mind-body therapies (meditation, guided imagery, and biofeedback), and tai chi/Qi Gong. While these less traditional methods are not normally designed to replace standard medical protocols, they may very well enhance their effectiveness by giving patients the ability and agency to experiment and select healing tools that are often self-administered and used in less stigmatizing nonclinical environments (Barrett, 2003).

As the VA has launched over 80 major studies of CIH methods among combat trauma survivors and the military has deployed training to help mitigate the impact of combat stress prior to traumatic experiences, the shift to include these asset-based treatments along with traditional evidence-based ones has broad implications on the manner of mitigating the costs of war. To appreciate the value of integrating a CIH perspective, this afterword is divided into three overall parts. The first section explores the limits of traditional pharmacological and psychoanalytic approaches to combat trauma. After we explore the current menu of traditional evidence-based treatments for the invisible wounds of war, we address their very significant limitations. Aside from the significant risk of abuse of prescription narcotics, a major difficulty is the widespread, uninformed perception among military members that mental health treatment will not benefit them. This has much to do with the culture of military service, which is pervasive and entrenched. To address this concern, the second section explains treatment stigma issues within warrior culture that impact care-seeking and self-care behaviors for both active military and veterans. Intelligently offering CIH to these populations requires understanding psychosocial influences. Finally, we explore CIH treatments and recommends scalable delivery platforms, reviewing current efforts within the VA system and discussing best practices and future research areas for implementation with active duty servicemembers.

CURRENT TREATMENTS AND THEIR LIMITATIONS

Poor mental health is a major health problem in the military veteran community, with estimated rates of stress injury and depression varying from 15 to 50 percent and incidence rates exceeding those in the civilian population (Acosta, Adamson, Farmer, Farris, & Feeney, 2014; Coughlin,

2012; Wilcox, Finnery, & Cedarbaum, 2013). Variance in the rate of depression reported in studies of veterans has been observed partly because depression in veterans is often undiagnosed (Thomas et al., 2015). Closely correlated with suicide, mental health issues place a servicemember at risk (Bossarte, 2013; Hoge & Castro, 2012). Military deployment to a war zone may elevate the risk of long-term physical, psychological, and social problems and reduce overall health status (Spelman, Hunt, Seal, & Burgo-Black, 2012), but its not an easy predictor of whether a veteran will struggle with mental health issues. Not everyone exposed to trauma or combat suffer from reactivity issues afterward, and many mental health issues are not causally linked to trauma. Among younger veterans of Iraq and Afghanistan, the greatest predictor of suicide is not deployment, but rather a recent separation from service (Friedman, 2015). Reintegration into new roles and loss of community felt when leaving the military contribute to depression among recently discharged veterans (Brenner & Barnes, 2012).

The Medical Model

Studying mental health can be a complicated process, as symptoms manifest on multiple levels and vary greatly from one diagnosed patient to the next (Hoge, 2010). Even the words used to describe the symptoms vary greatly. Professionals discussing the same stress injury symptoms may refer to post-traumatic stress (PTS), the more-stigmatizing post-traumatic stress disorder (PTSD), "stress reaction," "battle fatigue," or "operational stress." These trauma and stress disorder diagnoses are often accompanied by symptoms of depression in varying degrees of severity, and this co-occurrence may or may not be understood, recognized, and diagnosed (Hoge & Castro, 2012).

Conversations in the health-care field on the topic of behavioral medicine focus on the ways in which pharmacology and high-tech interventions drive social norms and attitudes about the role of individual agency in health outcomes (Seaward, 2004; Snyderman, 2014). The issue is as much economic as personal; chronic health conditions consume more than 75 percent of health-care expenditures, with health-care costs accounting for over 18 percent of the Gross National Product (GNP) (Department of Veterans Affairs, 2016a). Treatment for conditions, mental, physical, or both, often begin at secondary or even tertiary prevention levels, increasing cost and decreasing the likelihood of success. (Snyderman, 2013). Snyderman and Yoediono (2006) have proposed a prospective care model, utilizing a strategic personalized health plan and large health databases, including bio-psycho-social-genetic information to anticipate potential disease states and to allow for less costly prevention and early intervention.

Protocols within the Current Standard of Care

Currently, providers offer evidence-based treatments to patients that include the following: Cognitive Behavioral Therapy (CBT), Prolonged Exposure Therapy (PET), Dialectical Behavioral Therapy (DBT), Motivational Interviewing (MI), Eye movement desensitization and reprocessing (EMDR), and Acceptance and Commitment Therapy (ACT). Table 1 displays descriptions for each of the aforementioned treatments.

While the mental health treatment protocols discussed in Table 1 have shown promise in some studies (Hiraoka, Cook, Bivona, Meyer, & Morissette, 2016), documented limitations fuel the debate regarding the efficacy of these approaches. Beyond the fact that many studies of these protocols have been conducted with limited samples (Herbert et al., 2017) and with instruments that have not been psychometrically adapted for the psychologically traumatized veteran population (Kehle-Forbes et al., 2016), research has shown that veterans rarely volunteer participation in these mental health treatments, and when they do, dropout rates are high (Kehle-Forbes, Meis, Spoont, & Polusny, 2015).

Furthermore, Solomon and Heide (2005) stated that trauma victims often experience symptoms such as, but not limited to, irritability, heightened perceptions of danger, and difficulty with concentration—all of which are not alleviated by top-down trauma processing techniques such as Cognitive Behavioral Therapy. In contrast, bottom-up trauma processing approaches—which rely on biologically informed mind-body methods—such as Somatic Experiencing and Body Oriented Psychotherapy, permit traumatized patients to assign new meanings to events that are contaminated with painful feelings (Levine, 2010). Despite their demonstrated effectiveness, biologically informed treatment approaches have been absent from the standard menu of mental health therapies (Rankin, 2013).

Relying on pharmacological approaches to treatment has proven extremely problematic for patients in general and for military personnel in particular (Spelman et al. 2012). Unintentional overdose deaths parallel per capita sales of opioid analgesics. Overdose has become the leading cause of injury deaths among 25–65-year-olds, which is of particular concern in our veteran population (Centers for Disease Control and Prevention, 2017; Coughlin, 2012). The co-occurrence of mental health conditions such as post-traumatic stress disorder (PTSD), major depressive disorder (MDD) with alcohol and substance use has been linked to increased risk

Table 1   Descriptions of Current Mental Health Treatment Protocols

Treatment	Description[a]	Source
Cognitive Behavioral Therapy (CBT)	The class of interventions that are based on the basic premise that emotional disorders are maintained by cognitive factors and that psychological treatment leads to changes in these factors through cognitive (cognitive restructuring) and behavioral (e.g., exposure, behavioral experiments, relaxation training, social skills training) techniques.	Hofmann & Smits, 2008, p. 621
Prolonged Exposure Therapy (PET)	The overall aim of PET is to help trauma survivors emotionally process their traumatic experiences in order to diminish post-traumatic stress disorder (PTSD) and other trauma-related symptoms. The name "prolonged exposure" reflects the fact that the treatment program emerged from the long tradition of exposure therapy for anxiety disorders, in which clients are helped to confront safe but anxiety-evoking situations in order to overcome their excess fear and anxiety.	Foa, Hembree, & Rothbaum, 2007, p. 1
Eye Movement Desensitization and Reprocessing (EMDR)	Some Department of Veterans Affairs (VA) Medical Centers currently provide EMDR, an evidence-based therapy already supported by the Veterans Health Administration (VHA). Numerous studies have provided evidence for the efficacy of eye movement desensitization and reprocessing therapy (EMDR) in the treatment of PTSD, including recent studies showing it to be more efficient than traditional talk therapies (Davidson & Parker, 2001). The process pays attention to the stress response and brain reactivity of traumatized patients, working to decondition overactive synaptic firings. Repetitive redirecting of attention in EMDR induces a neurobiological state optimally configured to support the cortical integration of traumatic memories into general semantic networks and re-wire the brain after trauma. This can reduce reactivity to traumatic memories and shrink the overactive amygdala seen in patients with stress injuries (Stickgold, 2002).	Davidson & Parker, 2001; Stickgold, 2002

(continued)

Table 1   (continued)

Treatment	Description[a]	Source
Dialectical Behavioral Therapy (DBT)	DBT attends to five functions of comprehensive treatment: capability enhancement (skills training), motivational enhancement (individual behavioral treatment plans), generalization (in vivo assignments, phone consultation), structuring of the environment (programmatic emphasis on reinforcement of sobriety and adaptive behaviors), and capability and motivational enhancement of therapists (therapist team consultation group). The treatment has two major characteristics: a behavioral, problem-solving focus blended with acceptance-based strategies and an emphasis on dialectical processes.	Linehan et al., 2002, p. 14
Motivational Interviewing (MI)	MI is a directive, client-centered counseling style for eliciting behaviour change by helping clients to explore and resolve ambivalence. The strategies of motivational interviewing are more persuasive than coercive, more supportive than argumentative, and the overall goal is to increase the client's intrinsic motivation so that change arises from within rather than being imposed from without.	Rubak, Sandbaek, Lauritzen, & Christensen, 2005, p. 305
Acceptance and Commitment Therapy (ACT)	ACT is based on the view that many maladaptive behaviors are produced by unhealthy attempts to avoid or suppress thoughts, feelings, or bodily sensations. Among other components, patients are taught to (a) identify and abandon internally oriented control strategies, (b) accept the presence of difficult thoughts or feelings, (c) learn to "just notice" the occurrence of these private experiences, without struggling with them, arguing with them, or taking them to be literally true, and (d) focus on overt behaviors that produce valued outcomes.	Bach & Hayes 2002, p. 1130

[a] Descriptions are direct quotes from the sources listed in column 3.

for suicidality (Ohayan & Schatzberg, 2003). All of these disorders are associated with high-dose opioid utilization (Clark, 2004).

It is important to manage pain safely and effectively because chronic pain is the most common cause of work disability. In fact, more than 50 percent of male VA patients in primary care report chronic pain (Chapman, Lehman, Elliott, & Clark, 2006). The prevalence may be even higher in women veterans (Department of Veterans Affairs, 2014). The ramifications of overuse of pharmaceuticals to treat pain and often co-occurring mental health conditions have become widely understood, which has encouraged the VA to begin incorporating pain treatment plans that include the following behavioral medicine foci: patient lifestyle improvements (e.g., exercise, weight loss), support or education groups, physiotherapy modalities (e.g., physical therapy, occupational therapy, orthotics), and complementary and alternative therapies (Department of Veterans Affairs, 2016b). This emphasis on complementary modalities has proven uniquely successful for pain management (Denneson, Corson, & Dobscha, 2011). "Nonpharmacological treatment strategies are effective and should be an integral part of treatment for Veterans with pain" (Department of Veterans Affairs, 2014, p. 4). Most VA hospitals offer some type of complementary and integrative health approaches (Strauss, Lang, & Schnurr, 2017). According to internal VA memos, "The type of services offered at each site may depend on the need at that particular location" (Department of Veterans Affairs, 2016b, p. 1). VA directives will eventually inform VA sites about the approaches they must offer, as well as provide lists of approaches that are allowed to be offered within the Veterans Health Administration (VHA), based on the level of evidence. Sites will select from that list, depending on veteran demands at its location. Later in this chapter, the predictors of demand are discussed.

For the reasons highlighted above, the current clinical recovery paradigm is limited, and co-occurrence of pain issues or sleep disorders makes mental health service delivery more complex for veteran service providers (Chapman et al., 2006; Dobscha, Corson, Flores, Tansill, & Gerrity, 2008). Most veterans are not excited about embracing patient identities and accepting diagnoses (Malmin, 2013; Thomas, 2016).

Cultural Concerns

In some ways, the medical community's focus on access to psychotherapeutic treatment protocols represents progress. Stress injury and depression are real, and prior to Vietnam, they were often discussed as nothing more than cowardice or moral failure (Bossarte, 2013; Hoge, 2010). In other ways, a myopically focused treatment narrative sets up stereotype expectations of brokenness in the public consciousness. Standard medical approaches also ask the veterans to rely on external means (therapeutic and pharmaceutical interventions) to manage a chronic condition. Such an approach is anathema to cultural norms for veterans. Warrior subculture tends to promote the belief that acknowledging emotional pain is synonymous with weakness and, specifically, that asking for help for emotional distress or problems is unacceptable (Malmin, 2013). Depressed veterans face inexorable stigma when it comes to care-seeking for a possible or confirmed condition because of the normative values held within the warrior subculture (Thomas, 2016).

Culture is an important factor that shapes individual behavior through customized sets of attitudes, beliefs, and values shared by a large population (Shiraev & Levy, 2010). One's surrounding social norms play a vital role in shaping the attitudes and beliefs (Ajzen, 1991) commonly used to delineate and define culture. In insular communities, normative values can become highly prescriptive and are enforced in a myriad of intangible ways. Emotional norms become disciplinary tools, rendered more effective in communities with high levels of adherence to hierarchy (Ahmed, 2010). Especially in military communities that promote collectivism, this allows the expectations of others to weigh heavily on warriors' shoulders. The culture emphasizes being a functional member of the group who is able to perform his or her duties. Being labeled as inadequate leads to marginalization because the consequences of failure are so great; not competently performing said duties may lead to injury or death for others. The result of such a firmly entrenched value system is shame associated with patient-identity and mental health conditions (Thomas et al., 2016).

Within the military community, screening for depressive disorders and accessing medical care available to servicemembers suffering from depression are not the primary barriers to outcome improvement. Rather, the problem is getting veterans to avail themselves of treatment services (Currier, Holland, & Allen, 2012; Elnitsky et al., 2013; Koo & Maguen, 2014). In one post-deployment study, 42 percent of screened Reserve and National Guard soldiers answered questions in such a way that they were flagged as being in need of evaluations and possible treatment. However, only half of those soldiers referred sought that treatment for which they were referred. Only 30 percent of those that sought treatment adhered to the protocol, meaning that they followed the basic program in question through the full eight sessions (Coughlin, 2012; Greden et al., 2010). Similar treatment avoidance issues and low treatment-adherence rates are found in active-duty populations (Hoge, 2010).

Part of the issue is the cultural drift (Taylor, 2011) or the stated disconnect that military veterans feel from civilians, even civilian mental health professionals who treat the military population (Seal et al., 2009; Squier

Kraft, 2007). Servicemembers and veterans often feel they are wasting their time dealing with people who cannot relate to their perspective, and they may actually feel more comfortable in the war zone (Hoge, 2010). Qualitative studies have shown that veterans self-report (a) a sense of burdensomeness and extreme disconnect from civilians post-service and (b) feelings linked to a failed sense of belonging and desire for death (Ilgen et al., 2012; Tanielan & Jaycox, 2008). Studies focused specifically on racial minority and female veterans found that these descriptions of symptoms and feelings of disconnect were markedly similar, though more pronounced and likely to be of greater severity (Duhart, 2012; Gutierrez et al., 2013).

Clinicians generally agree that it can be tough to get military personnel in their doors the first time, and harder still to keep a patient coming back for a full course of traditional mental health treatment (Greden et al., 2010). For this reason, professional discussions about healing war-traumatized veterans cannot be limited to psychotherapy treatment protocols (Thomas, 2016). Veterans often reject patient identities, creating a major barrier to mental health care within this population even when comprehensive services with current standards of care are being offered and are made discreetly available (Hoge, 2010; Malmin, 2013). The current medical model in the United States and in the VA asks veterans struggling emotionally to label a problem and identify it as being in need of some sort of help. Professionals use diagnostic labels like PTSD or major depression to mark a veteran as permanently disabled (Held & Owens, 2013). This paradigm is shifting, particularly in the VA, as the VA medical staff embraces the Patient Centered Care model noted later in the writing.

Without the ability to realize their own agency in selecting and implementing healing protocols, many veterans who need treatment will not seek it because they believe themselves powerless and weak in the process. Through a review of self-reported opinions about mental health, one study reviewing a national sample of veterans, some involved with the VA health system and some not, showed that cultural prohibition against traditional care-seeking among veterans was a significant barrier to care (Thomas et al., 2015). Only 2 percent of over fifty-four thousand veteran respondents (already service-separated) thought clinical mental health treatment was a helpful service that could help a person live a normal, happy life. Interestingly, researchers found that stigma could be overcome with exposure and experience; if a veteran had a diagnosis and had been working with a mental health provider, they were 24 times more likely to have a positive opinion about what mental health treatment could do for a person than a veteran who had not. Once they were in the door, opinions changed, but few ever opened the door (Thomas et al., 2015). These data point to an overwhelming need for care providers to meet veterans where they are and to speak culturally competent language when reaching out (Malmin, 2013). Any programming that doesn't stem from an assets-based perspective or that which requires a patient identity will miss too many recalcitrant veterans who need to be, but will never opt in as, participants (Thomas & Albright, 2018). To combat suicide rates and promote military and veteran mental health, a new approach is required, one that embraces peer education, physical agency, and individual effort (Kobau et al., 2011; Seaward, 2004). With exposure to a series of alternatives for the promotion of healing and well-being, traditional health-care providers may be able to dislodge veterans and military members from a limiting mindset about help-seeking and treatment plan adherence.

COMPLEMENTARY CARE—A PATIENT-CENTERED APPROACH

The evidence base for somatic protocols is well established; there is significant amount of rigorously conducted research on trauma therapies that emphasize breath, body, and complementary practice (Jha & Kiyonaga, 2010; Jha, Stanley, Kiyanoga, Wong, & Gelfand, 2010; van der Kolk, 2014). Neuroscience is contributing to the evidence building to support the importance of CIH protocols in the treatment of trauma. Stephen Porges' Polyvagal Theory highlights the ways in which all humans constantly check for safety at an unconscious level, especially in social relationships. For those traumatized, it is imperative that they feel safe, in mind and body, before healing can happen (Porges, 2011). Calming the body and mind through CIH allows for this (Diamond, Campbell, Park, Halonen, & Zoladz, 2007). Traumatic memory fragments are not easily retrieved through the rational brain, but are instead experienced through intense emotions, physical sensations, and images. Talking is not effective in reaching these memories, but sensing the body is (van der Kolk, 2014). Interpersonal neurobiology explains the interrelationship of the endocrine system and nervous system by outlining the role of mirror neurons in attachment and bodily memory (Siegel and Solomon, 2003). The development of understanding of the brain's default network and the present centered network offers neurological explanation for patient-reported benefits to somatic interventions (Andrews-Hanna, Smallwood, & Spreng, 2014).

Mindfulness interventions have been highlighted in community setting studies as effective in reducing stress and anxiety and in individual case studies looking at mindfulness and mood recovery (Jouper & Johansson, 2012). The Department of Defense has seen the validity of yoga in Wounded

Warrior recovery programs, and it is slowly expanding research partnerships and building the population-specific evidence base. Studies on one particular yoga *nidra* protocol (a form of body-focused meditation, called iRest®) at Walter Reed yielded positive qualitative feedback and resulted in a three-week version being included in the treatment program at the deployment clinic (Hoge et al., 2008). Women veterans have responded well to such interventions; another study of iRest utilized in an eight-week program with women surviving military sexual trauma (MST) found statistical reductions in PTSD, depression, and negative thoughts of self-blame (Pence, Katz, Huffman, & Cojucar, 2014).

Comparative research examining somatic protocols and traditional therapies has noted non-inferiority in the somatic practices (Hendricks, Turner, & Hunt, 2014; van der Kolk, 2014). In particular, yoga interventions have been useful for people with stress-related illnesses. A 2007 study charted the self-reported quality of life improvements in two groups of physically healthy participants currently participating in Cognitive Behavioral Therapy (CBT) for stress-related anxiety. The yoga program primarily focused on postures and breathwork and cognitive therapy only on individual sessions with a therapist. Each program included 10 sessions over four months. Participants in both groups showed significant improvements in both psychological (self-rated stress and stress behavior, anger, exhaustion, quality of life) and physiological (blood pressure, heart rate, salivary cortisol) outcomes. There was no significant difference between groups, but the group incorporating yoga into their routine reported significantly higher quality of life indicators (Granath, Ingvarsson, von Thiele, & Lundberg, 2006).

In the traditional treatment sector, somatic protocols fit well within military culture and permit veterans to seek treatment without the patient identity designation (van der Kolk & Macfarlane, 2012). Cultural competency means not only trying to understand the veteran experience but also learning the most effective ways to communicate with different subsets of the veteran and military populations. Health professionals working to treat mental health problems such as depression and stress illness must understand the confluence of warrior culture and mental health issues in the veteran community and design healing protocols that offer relief in a form veterans can accept.

Even though, as noted above, there is rigorous evidence, many studies of CIH have small sample sizes and lower methodological rigor, often due to funding issues. That is changing with the veterans' request for alternatives to traditional therapies and the positive trend of the CIH studies. Currently, the VA's Office of Health Services Research and Development (HSRD) has over eighty ongoing research projects studying various somatic modalities (Department of Veterans Affairs, 2016a).

Somatic Protocols in Detail

What potentially applicable complementary and integrative modalities exist? We've divided them into two categories. First, we reviewed protocols with demonstrated potential for inclusion in existing VHA psychological service offerings that can be offered by current clinicians. In a number of VHA psychotherapy practices, these are already in practice offerings. We also reviewed newer/niche modalities that might be more effectively provided by people other than clinicians, operating as adjuncts and partners at VHA facilities. Some of these niche offerings are already offered at VHAs that believe in their utility, often brought in with partner organizations staffed by volunteers.

Potential (and actual) clinician-offered options include the following:

- Acceptance and Commitment Therapy (ACT): ACT incorporates principles of mindfulness and encourages participants to focus on behavior that is in accordance with their values and purpose (Hayes, Masuda, Bissett, Luoma, & Guerrero, 2004). Clinicians using ACT attempt to interrupt psychopathology caused by unbalanced attempts to control feelings, thoughts, and memories. Emphasis is placed on altering patterns of present-moment avoidance and lack of clarity about what life values are and congruent actions. There is an emphasis on feeling emotions in the body sans judgment and ultimately choosing active behaviors that are in alignment with personal values. Preliminary research on ACT's effectiveness indicates that it is helpful in reducing anxiety, depressive symptoms (Forman, Herbert, Moitra, Yeomans, & Geller, 2007), opiate abuse (Hayes, Wilson, et al., 2004), and the re-hospitalization rate of patients with psychosis. This evidence-based therapy is already supported and delivered by VHA.

- Somatic Experiencing (SE) and Sensorimotor Psychotherapy: Somatic Experiencing (Payne, Levine, & Crane-Godreau, 2015) and Sensorimotor Psychotherapy (Langmuir, Kirsh, & Classen, 2012; Ogden & Fisher, 2015) were developed by psychotherapists in an effort to utilize movements of the body to unlock stored memories and thwarted movements of the body that could not be processed at the time of the trauma. SE is a form of trauma therapy that emphasizes guiding the client's attention to interoceptive, kinesthetic, and proprioceptive experiences. Such inner attention, in addition to the use of kinesthetic and interoceptive imagery, can lead to the resolution of symptoms resulting from chronic and traumatic stress by calming self-protective and defensive responses or of stress reactivity by creating space for the discharge and regulation of excess autonomic arousal (Payne et al., 2015).

- Progressive Muscle Relaxation: Progressive Muscle Relaxation (PMR) was developed in therapeutic settings to relax the body before talk therapy by controlled tightening of muscles in directed order (Seaward, 2004). A study of a single session large group progressive muscle relaxation intervention on stress reduction found significant reductions in stress (Rausch, Gramling, & Auerbach, 2006). PMR was found in a study of eight VA PTSD treatment programs to be the third-most popular CAM treatment (Libby, Pilver, & Desai, 2012).

- Meditation (Mantram Repetition, mindfulness practices, Mindfulness Based Stress Reduction [MBSR], contemplative prayer, Heartmath®, iRest®, Transcendental Meditation [TM], *vipassana*): These can easily be brought into group therapy or individual therapy settings. There is a rapidly growing pool of research on the benefits of meditation (Hempel et al., 2014). The benefits of meditation have been studied with active military (Barnes, Monto, Williams, & Rigg, 2016; Johnson et al., 2014) and veterans (Heffner, Crean, & Kemp, 2016). A 2012 review found that mindfulness and meditation in general were the most utilized CAM treatments in PTSD treatment programs. A mantram repetition program has been developed, trained for, and disseminated throughout VA, and a randomized trial on veterans had showed clinically meaningful improvements in PTSD symptoms over treatment as usual (Bormann, Thorp, Wetherell, Golshan, & Lang, 2013).

- Energy Medicine: The Emotional Freedom Technique (tapping) utilizes the calming effects of engaging acupuncture points while presently experiencing and resolving the sensorial results of an upsetting event (Church, 2013). Controlled trials with veterans diagnosed with PTSD have showed statistically significant results (Church et al., 2013).

- Breathwork: Evidence for controlled breath practices has demonstrated that participants can reduce self-reported stress levels, lower blood pressure and heart rate, relax muscles and experience sounder sleep, decrease anxiety, have less pain, improve immune function, and have better concentration. Breathing practices can include abdominal diaphragmatic breathing, ocean sounding breath (Ujayi), alternate nostril breathing, three-part breath, and bee breath (Department of Defense, 2017). In a randomized controlled longitudinal study, it was found that PTSD and anxiety symptoms in veterans were reduced with a breathing protocol (Seppälä et al., 2014).

- Guided Imagery (GI): A form of meditation, GI has been effective in addressing PTSD symptoms of hyperarousal, intrusion, and constriction and the core experiences of disempowerment and disconnection in both individual and group sessions. The GI process allows access to subconscious feelings, images, and memories and fosters empowerment and reconnection through self-understanding and an alliance with the therapist. Guided Imagery and Music (GIM) was successfully utilized to lower PTSD scores with Vietnam Veterans in a psychiatric setting (Blake & Bishop, 1994). GI is the fourth most popular CAM modality utilized in studied VA PTSD treatment programs (Libby et al., 2012).

Specialized, adjunct health professionals can (and some already) provide the following:

- Acupuncture and self-administered acupressure: Acupuncturists utilize needles or heated cups to move stuck energy in the body. Acupressure is the process of applying pressure to acupuncture points to achieve similar results as acupuncture. Acupuncture can provide relief from pain (Hempel et al., 2013). Battlefield acupuncture is being taught in VA currently to relieve acute pain. It is used in theater currently by the U.S. military (Niemtzow, Belard, & Nogier, 2015).

- Nutritional Therapy: Nutrition is an incredibly underutilized mode of creating wellness, as proper food intake has been linked to better mental health outcomes (Institute of Medicine (IOM), 2011; Seaward, 2004). The VA has a Nutrition and Food Services Office, and its benefits might be greater when seen as part of the whole health perspective.

- Spiritual Fitness: Chaplains in the service of VA can be an incredible resource in working through moral injury (Drescher et al., 2011). An important piece of working through moral injury is letting go of a victim mentality, blame and shame, and forgiveness of self and others (Nash, 2010). Protocols addressing moral injury as separate and distinct from stress injuries are starting to be implemented in some VA service networks as understandings of the different conditions improve through study and provider experience (Gray et al., 2012; Wood, 2016). Spiritual practices or religious therapies were the seventh most utilized modality in VA PTSD programs as of 2012 (Libby et al., 2012).

- Physical Yoga (including breathing practices): A mindful movement practice that has proven popular with veterans in adaptive, clinical, and fitness settings, yoga's benefits for pain management, mental health, stress reduction, and attention or focus improvement are backed by research (Hendricks et al., 2014). In particular, yoga interventions have been useful for people with stress-related illnesses when compared to traditional talk therapies (Raingruber & Robinson, 2007). One study directly compared the self-reported quality of life improvements in two groups of physically healthy participants currently participating in Cognitive Behavioral Therapy (CBT) for stress-related anxiety. The intervention group continued the therapy and participated in an intervention based on meditation and physical yoga. The control group continued their regimen of CBT. The group incorporating yoga into their routine reported significantly higher quality of life indicators. Yoga was the sixth most popular modality utilized in VA PTSD treatment programs as of 2012 (Libby et al., 2012).

- Massage Therapy and Self-Massage Methods: Releasing tension in the body has been linked to mental health outcome improvements; during such therapy, patients often report cathartic releases on the massage table (Walach, Güthlin, & König, 2003). The patient feels physical relief from the pain of stored tension and loosening of muscles that pull the body out of alignment (Sherman, Dixon, Thompson, & Cherkin, 2006). In a study of the available research regarding massage, high-quality studies were found that noted the potential benefits of massage on pain; however, the strength of the research was less than moderate (Miake-Lye et al., 2016). Massage was offered in a pilot program of female veterans with PTSD and chronic pain. It was found that the intimate touch was tolerated by this population (Price, McBride, Hyerle, & Kivlahan, 2007).

- Tai Chi: Tai chi is a slow-moving martial art, and its purpose is to enhance internal balance and energy, or "qi" (Meeks & Jeste, 2009). Originating in China around 500 BC, tai chi consists of a series of forms and movements that involve gentle and slow motions. It has been used to decrease symptoms of depression, insomnia, and stress (Chi, Jordan-Marsh, Guo, Xie, & Bai, 2013; Meeks & Jeste, 2009). Lee, Lee, and Woo (2009) also report that health-related quality of life improved with tai chi in a population of nursing home residents. A systemic review of the research on tai chi was conducted by the VA Evidence Synthesis Program of the Health Services Research and Development, and it noted statistically significant outcomes from tai chi for hypertension, fall prevention, and cognitive performance (Solloway et al., 2016).

- Healing Touch and Reiki: These techniques involve touch or practitioner's presence to move the energy of the patient with the intent of easing pain or promoting relaxation. Reiki was developed in Japan (VanderVaart, Gijsen, de Wildt, & Koren, 2009). Healing touch evolved from the energetic healing capacity of Janet Mentgen, RN, in the 1980s by the American Holistic Nurses Association (Anderson & Taylor, 2011). A randomized controlled trial of the use of healing touch with guided imagery for PTSD in returning Iraq and Afghanistan veterans found clinically and statistically significant reductions in PTSD symptoms as well as depression and an increase in the mental quality of life (Jain et al., 2012). A case study documented the results of healing touch sessions on seven veterans, noting a wide range of positive results for patients with spinal cord injuries (Wardell, Rintala, & Tan, 2008).

- Movement therapies are multimodal and are popular mental and physical healing options. Methods include the Alexander method (Furlan et al., 2011; Little et al., 2008), the Egoscue method (Egoscue & Gittines, 2014), the Feldenkrais method (Bearman & Shafarman, 1999; Öhman, Åström, & Malmgren-Olsson, 2011), and Pilates (Lim, Poh, Low, & Wong, 2011; Pereira et al., 2012). These movement techniques utilize slow, mindful movements to impact specific misalignments and weaknesses within the body and are well combined with physical therapy. Programs for wounded veterans have proven popular (Bowman, 2015).

- Animal Therapy: Service animals and therapy animals can accompany the veterans to reduce stress reactivity and mitigate stress injury symptoms such as flashbacks. Dogs and horses are commonly used for service animal treatments, and evaluation results with veteran patients report positive responses to program participation (Cantin & Marshall-Lucette, 2011; Cumella & Simpson, 2014).

- Aromatherapy: Aromatherapy involves the use of scents to calm, or invigorate, the mind and body. Essential oils are often used to impact the olfactory senses to stimulate the body's relaxation response (Cooke & Ernst, 2000).

- Biofeedback: Biofeedback utilizes sensors to measure the physical phenomena of stress or relaxation, such as the heart rate, temperature and moisture of the skin, heart rate variability (Chalmers, Quintana, Abbott, & Kemp, 2014), and brain waves. Some sensors can be easily transported and can be used with a smart phone or small hand-held device (Henriques, Keffer, Abrahamson, & Horst, 2011). Biofeedback was listed as eighth most popular CIH in 2012 in VA PTSD programs (Libby et al., 2012).

- Drumming: Drumming is an ancient form of music that involves hitting a drum skin or drum head with one's hand or a stick. It has been used as a form of music therapy with Vietnam veterans (Burt, 1995), patients with anger problems (Slotoroff, 1994), trauma (Bensimon, Amir, & Wolf, 2008), substance abuse (Winkelman, 2003), and a variety of psychiatric illnesses (Longhofer & Floersch, 1993). There are also physical benefits of drumming such as decreased stress, increased immune functioning, and improved cardiovascular health (Bittman et al., 2001). A drum circle can foster veterans' creativity and cohesion by teaching them a unique form of expression that can be a very cathartic medium. Bensimon et al. (2008) found that it helped to reduce the symptoms of PTSD and also create a sense of openness and cohesion.

- Health Coaching: It is the process of mentoring and providing wellness wisdom as well as working with veterans to help them feel their best through use of the Whole Health Plan (Department of Veterans Affairs, 2016b). Instead of prescribing one diet or way of exercising, health coaches tailor individualized wellness programs to meet veterans' needs. There is an intensive health coaching course available to VHA employees (Collins et al., 2015).

- Somatic Protocols: These can be used to help veterans develop coping skills to prepare for intensive trauma work, and they can offer a place to release emotions and enhance the ability to create positive emotions. Somatic protocols can also be used during traditional Western trauma sessions to bring out suppressed issues (Emerson, Hopper, & LeVine, 2011), and they can be utilized as an adjunct to process what came up during traditional sessions (van der Kolk, 2014). There is a caveat regarding the use of somatic protocols among veterans: sometimes veterans use them, such as traditional group talk therapy, to avoid emotions and trauma work. For example, sometimes veterans will take mindfulness classes indefinitely but avoid processing their trauma. They receive benefits of relaxation, but do not address the reason they need to relax (Becker, 2008).

Current VHA Initiatives to Deliver CIH

One of the challenges in the liberal distribution of complementary modalities among veterans often involves licensure. VHA facilities generally hire licensed professionals to work directly with patients (Department of Veterans Affairs, 2016a). As complementary modalities establish national licensure programs (a slow process), they are more likely to be integrated in patient care systems. Consider the following update regarding chiropractic care, a licensed modality in the United States, from VA: "Chiropractic care is offered to Veterans throughout the VHA as a rehabilitative service that is part of the Medical Benefits Package for Veterans and thus available system-wide to all Veterans" (Department of Veterans Affairs, 2016a).

CIH practitioners rarely possess formal, federally recognized licensure. They practice under certification requisites in alignment with their specific community standard of care and scope of practice. Field standardization will help with rollout, though the research basis for practice utility is broad already (Seaward, 2004; Thomas & Plummer Taylor, 2015). While individual VA Medical Centers (VAMCs) can evaluate well-being instructors for local needs, national standards would provide direction, structure, and reduction of liability. To that end, certain professional organizations, such as the International Association of Yoga Therapists (IAYT), have begun the process of creating professional certification requirements to which VA can look for professional ethics and minimum requirements, training, and expectations (International Association of Yoga Therapists, 2017). Licensure may come later.

In 2014, researchers conducted a project to better understand the factors that facilitated or hindered new modality implementation in VAMCs (Taylor et al., 2019). They found that organizing the individual types of CIH into one program instead of individually integrating them into departments and getting leadership support (with a CIH strategic plan and steering committee) helped medical centers implement CIH. Additionally, enthusiastic and capable adjunct instructors made the implementation process more feasible. Common CIH adoption or implementation challenges reported included difficulties in hiring CIH practitioners; difficulties in coding/documenting CIH use; insufficient or inconsistent CIH funding; insufficient or inappropriate space to deliver CIH; lack of CIH practitioners' time; and confusion about employment of CIH providers without standard/recognized occupational codes, position descriptions, or credentialing criteria. Overall, the research team found that respondents indicated a need for CIH practices to be formalized to make implementation easier (Taylor et al., 2019).

In one study, it was noted that military personnel reported using CIH practices between two and seven times the rate of civilian patients, most frequently choosing prayer (24%), massage (14%), and relaxation techniques (11%) such as meditation or movement practice (Goertz et al., 2013). Veterans recently returning from deployment use integrative techniques as predicted by certain health issues, stress levels, race, age, gender, education, and income, which are also the determining factors for the utilization of the CIH modalities (Park, Finkelstein-Fox, Barnes, Mazure, & Hoff, 2016). Variables including education, gender, high stress levels, and high levels of military sexual trauma are predictors of higher levels of usage of CIH in general. Most popular modalities with newly transitioning veterans are massage, chiropractic, yoga, and acupuncture treatments (Park et al., 2016). This is quite different from the order of offerings in VA PTSD treatment programs (Libby et al., 2012). As the DOD and VA move forward with CIH, it will be important to clearly understand the demographics and psychosocial characteristics of the population such treatments beyond the standard of care are intended to reach.

Of the modalities noted above, those that are more on the fringe and might pose additional concerns for acceptance among patients and health-care providers, in the authors' opinion, are energy medicine (which includes Emotionally Focused Therapy EFT, healing touch, and Reiki), tai chi, aromatherapy, and drumming. This is based on the more esoteric reasons that they are beneficial and are moving energy which impact the olfactory nerves, and therefore memories. However, depending on the demographics of the intended recipients of such programs and treatments, fringe status is not the best predictor of patient receptivity and popularity. Drumming, for example, has been well received by veteran participants as it is fun and social (Bittman et al., 2001). Rating the most controversial modalities from the perspective of the recipients will help planners consider timing and methods of introduction (Barrett, 2003).

SCALABLE DELIVERY: MAKING CIH AVAILABLE FOR VETERANS

Health professionals working to prevent and treat mental health problems such as depression and stress illness must understand the confluence of warrior culture and mental health issues in the veteran community (Thomas, 2016). Culturally informed somatic protocols would be best implemented in participatory fashion in the training environment rather than in treatment settings, but their role in existing treatment settings is vital nonetheless. To that end, VA is actively participating in research and development to work with VA leadership and health-care providers to transform VA's health system from the traditional medical model, which focuses on treating specific issues, "to a . . . model that promotes whole health for Veterans and their families" (Department of Veterans Affairs, 2017b).

The Office of Patient Centered Care and Cultural Transformation (OPCC&CT) was formed in 2011. Director Tracy Gaudet called for revolutionary change in the health-care system during the 2009 Summit on Integrative Medicine and the Health of the Public (Institute of Medicine, 2009), sparking a push to formalize exploration of nontraditional treatment protocols to maximize patient accessibility. Chronic conditions that are primarily driven by lifestyle choices and health behaviors account for 75 percent of the U.S. health-care costs, or approximately $1.87 trillion per year. The current system's disease-oriented, problem-focused design is ill-suited to address these significant chronic issues. Various pilots of new models of care are already in place and producing positive returns on investment, while providing better health outcomes (Institute of Medicine, 2009). The OPCC&CT was created to bring this necessary revolution to VA. It is focused on a Whole Health System model that incorporates physical care with psychosocial care focused on the veteran's personal health and life goals, aiming to provide personalized, proactive, patient-driven care through multidisciplinary teams of health professionals (Shulkin, 2016).

New practices appeal to many veterans, specifically when efforts are peer led (Thomas et al., 2015). The Whole Health System is founded on using peer specialists and health coaches. There were over one thousand peer specialists in VA's system in October 2015. A peer specialist is someone who is recovering from their own mental illness, who relates to and supports others going through their healing (Department of Veterans Affairs, 2017a).

The Integrative Health Coordinating Center (IHCC) is charged with increasing access to quality CIH treatments. Operating within the OPCC&CT, it aims to "support clinical standardization, business processes, policy development and the further expansion of these approaches throughout VA" (Department of Veterans Affairs, 2017b, p. 1). The CIH approaches that the IHCC will request VA facilities to offer include many mentioned in this chapter, which have strong, evidence-based support. All recommended approaches that will be included in the medical benefits package need to have evidence of safety and, at a minimum, promising or potential benefits (Department of Veterans Affairs, 2017b).

To pilot the Whole Health Model, in 2016 the OPCC&CT funded seven integrative care sites, and in 2017, they are funding 11 more. In Senate Bill 524, Section 933 of the Comprehensive Addiction and Recovery Act of 2016, Congress requires 15 diverse sites to pilot integrative care for three years. The network directors who manage the Veterans Integrated Service Networks (VISNs) have agreed to fund 18 sites (the same or different sites from those established in 2016 and 2017) for an additional three years. This will provide five years of data to determine what increase in quality of life and cost avoidance can be gained through integrative care and utilization of CIH. In a review of only two months of pilot data, the following were observed: improved physical and mental health symptoms, decreased medication use, and positive experiences and patient satisfaction (Department of Veterans Affairs, 2016b).

CIH providers often report when working with veteran patients that there is a great deal of variance in enthusiasm levels for the new treatment options (Department of Veterans Affairs, 2014; Pence et al. 2014). Many patients with depression, anxiety, and PTSD deal with isolation. Providing group support to build a network of friends and activities sufficient to sustain the veteran, given the importance of connection, would create foundational support from which to work through intensive therapies (Malmin, 2013). This support also creates the opportunity for the veteran to give back to the community and thereby increase a sense of meaning. In addition, readiness matters when engaging in behavioral health practices (Hendricks et al., 2014). To increase a feeling of receiving value, a tiered approach to providing services would serve the veteran and VA; as the Whole Health Model promotes, veterans must be agents in their own care plan creation. It would be effective and efficient if providers were supported in requiring that patients take motivational interviewing (MI; an evidence-based practice) before partaking in other services. During MI, the patients can become clear about whether it makes sense to invest their time in a treatment that will require personal investment, perhaps movement, and adherence to repetitive protocols. The benefits would also be explained.

Tailoring programs for relevance to resonate with veteran patients is needed. A need also exists for further research that explores the attitudes, beliefs, and opinions of veterans toward programming that is focused on resilience-building and post-traumatic growth (Tedeschi & Calhoun, 2004). The question of how to make behavioral medicine available, culturally competent, and appealing to different subpopulations of veterans is an important one; the advancement of veteran mental health could benefit tremendously from qualitative research, specifically case studies of successful programming (Coughlin, 2012). Rigorous program evaluations of culturally sensitive content, as well as the validation of program exemplars, which the VA has begun (Saenger, Duva, & Abraham, 2014), could facilitate the wide distribution and acceptance of somatic protocols aimed at improving veteran mental health outcomes (Thomas et al., 2016).

SCALABLE DELIVERY: MAKING CIH AVAILABLE FOR ACTIVE DUTY SERVICEMEMBERS

It is important to create programs aimed at post-service quality of life improvement and healing, but the biggest impacts can be made from a prevention angle (Thomas & Plummer Taylor, 2015). The reason for this is that stigma isn't going away, and we can reach more personnel while they are still serving than after they leave. The challenge for health professionals looking to stem the tide of service suicides and improve quality of life for veterans lies in shifting from a focus on problems toward a focus on capacity-building (Fletcher & Sarkar, 2013). In this space, there is massive opportunity to make a positive impact. Training protocols differ from treatment prescriptions, and they address the problem preventively, without the same stigma barriers (Foran, Adler, McGurk, & Bliese, 2012). These protocols are often best implemented in participatory fashion in the training environment, rather than in treatment settings (Thomas, Plummer Taylor, Hamner, Glazer, & Kaufman, 2015).

Pilot research conducted using somatic protocols to control the nervous system and increase working memory capacity has yielded interesting results (Vasterling et al., 2006). Working memory capacity contributes to emotional regulation as well as upper-level cognitive functioning, and more capacity is an indicator of increased psychological resilience (Jha, Stanley, & Baime, 2010). Researchers from the Mind-Fitness Training Institute conducted one such study on a company of U.S. Marines during pre-deployment work-ups, seeking to answer the question of whether a mindfulness based behavioral health intervention could improve the resilience of Marine Corps reservists preparing for a tour in Iraq and prevent depression problems after returning home. Attempting a mixed-methods approach to the explanatory and instrumental case study, the researchers studied one unit of 34 reservists in the pre-deployment work-up phase. In addition to the normal training required before heading overseas, these reservists underwent a carefully tailored yoga and mindfulness program designed to improve their ability to manage both chronic and acute traumatic stress. Results were statistically significant in the studied population, demonstrating that adherence to intervention protocol for 15 minutes each day noticeably improved working memory capacity (Stanley, Schaldach, Kiyonaga, & Jha, 2011).

Training active duty military personnel to regulate their nervous systems may actually prevent poor mental health outcomes before they become issues. Management of reactivity could be a performance enhancer for the active duty component. High stress reactivity and depression hinder the ability of servicemembers to perform complex missions and interact with foreign nationals. The modern battlefield involves interaction with civilians and allies as a matter of course. For example, research has shown that soldiers who screened positively for mental health problems were three times more likely to report having engaged in unethical behavior while being deployed (Teng et al., 2013). Behaviors ran the gamut from unnecessary property damage to noncombatant injury or harm, all diametrically opposed to the U.S. mission of winning hearts and minds. These issues leave behind moral injuries with which servicemembers may struggle well into their future (Wood, 2016).

Early efforts indicate that a peer-led model focusing on resiliency, somatic protocols, and performance enhancement works in the training sector and reduces overall stigma against performance enhancement practices because everyone participates. Perhaps the reason for the success of such programs lies in the fact that each program is led by a trusted informant, and no one has to take on a patient role to participate (Johnson et al., 2014). To train is to actively participate, a wellness concept with which servicemembers are already familiar. Framing mindfulness training and somatic protocols as a way to "bulletproof the brain" renders palatable a training opportunity designed to create more effective warriors with mental endurance; framing this as promotion of combat fitness, resilience, and mental endurance renders it accessible to the military population (Thomas & Albright, 2018). In the veteran population, training opportunities can be created by providing ongoing wellness opportunities and teaching somatic protocols that "bulletproof" and make the body, mind, and spirit resilient.

We have to speak the language of warriors when we talk about resiliency cultivation. By establishing mental fitness as another component of optimal combat readiness, we establish resiliency training as a crucial component of mission preparedness and remove the stigma of such practices for post-deployment troops who may be struggling with stress illnesses of varying degrees. The message can become directive; just as Marines and soldiers learn mission essential skills and train their bodies for arduous combat, we must adopt practices designed to train and promote health in the mind, body, and spirit in a holistic sense (Thomas & Albright, 2018).

When we consider how we could apply these basic recommendations to military veterans seeking relief from reintegration stress or to active duty military preparing for it, we must consider how to make stress management a testable metric. Biofeedback tools exist that can do this, and there is exciting future work standardizing a theoretically based, validated training curriculum and using an individual's ability to deescalate their nervous system response as a performance metric (Thomas & Albright, 2018). In this way, biofeedback testing will make CIH practices to improve resilience, a performance metric for the active duty component that will improve mental health outcomes for later veterans. The intent is to move self-awareness and resilience into trackable standards territory and motivate learning, training, practice, and performance in our community's culture (Thomas, 2016).

Checking for DHEA and blood cortisol ratios or conducting periodic blood cortisol checks can be as important as other physical standards are in the military (Jha, Stanley, & Bairme, 2010; Thomas & Plummer Taylor, 2015). Biomarkers tell us quickly whether someone is taking time to practice balanced wellness. The future is exciting from clinical, training, and prevention perspectives. It offers tremendous promise for future military personnel, who will be asked to embrace a holistic wellness training regimen to make them better at their jobs and more resilient in their lives, both during and after their service to our country.

APPENDIX A

Suggested Reading

RESILIENCE

- *The Upside of Stress: Why Stress Is Good for You, and How to Get Good at It*, by Kelly McGonigal
- *Trauma and Recovery: The Aftermath of Violence—from Domestic Abuse to Political Terror*, by Judith Herman, MD
- *Widen the Window: Training Your Brain and Body to Thrive during Stress and Recovery from Trauma*, by Elizabeth A. Stanley
- *Bulletproofing the Psyche: Preventing Mental Health Problems in Our Military and Veterans*, edited by Kate Hendricks Thomas and David L. Albright
- *A Mindful Nation: How a Simple Practice Can Help Us Reduce Stress, Improve Performance, and Recapture the American Spirit*, by Congressman Tim Ryan
- *Why Zebras Don't Get Ulcers: The Acclaimed Guide to Stress, Stress-Related Diseases, and Coping*, by Robert M. Sapolsky
- *The Body Keeps the Score: Brain, Mind, and Body in the Healing of Trauma*, by Bessel Van der Kolk

SELF-CARE

- *Eastern Body Western Mind: Psychology and the Chakra System as a Path to the Self,* by Anodea Judith
- *Atomic Habits: An Easy and Proven Way to Build Good Habits and Break Bad Ones,* by James Clear
- *Best Practices for Yoga with Veterans,* by the Yoga Service Council
- *Present Over Perfect: Leaving Behind Frantic for a Simpler, More Soulful Way of Living,* by Shauna Niequist
- *Just Roll with It Wellness Journal,* by Sarah Plummer Taylor and Kate Hendricks Thomas

SOCIAL SUPPORT

- *Tribe: On Homecoming and Belonging,* by Sebastian Junger
- *Love Sense: The Revolutionary New Science of Romantic Relationships,* by Dr. Sue Johnson

SPIRITUAL PRACTICE

- *Anatomy of the Spirit: The Seven Stages of Power and Healing,* by Carolyn Myss
- *Reinventing the Body, Resurrecting the Soul: How to Create a New You,* by Deepak Chopra
- *Of Mess and Moxie: Wrangling Delight Out of This Wild and Glorious Life,* by Jen Hatmaker
- *What Your Body Knows About God: How We Are Designed to Connect, Serve, and Thrive,* by Rob Moll
- *The Language of God: A Scientist Presents Evidence for Belief,* by Francis S. Collins

MILITARY CULTURAL COMPETENCE

- *Rule Number Two: Lessons from a Combat Hospital,* by Heidi Squier Kraft
- *What Have We Done: The Moral Injury of Our Longest Wars,* by David Wood
- *Once a Warrior, Always a Warrior,* by Charles Hoge

APPENDIX B

Breathwork and Meditation for
Integration, Balance, and Clarity

ALTERNATE NOSTRIL BREATHING

Background

Did you know that your nose is directly linked to your brain and your nervous system? We breathe predominantly through one nostril or the other at any given time. Take a few breaths in and out of your nose now and see what you notice. Is one nostril more open than the other? The dominant nostril alternates rhythmically every 90–150 minutes. The rhythm itself is mediated mainly through structures in the hypothalamus and pituitary, though other areas in the brain are also involved.

You may use the technique of inhaling and exhaling exclusively through either the left or right nostril in order to benefit from the quality associated with that nostril. Consciously using different breath ratios can yield varied effects. For instance, breathe exclusively through the left nostril to help you feel calm and to integrate unwanted negative emotions and stress. This exercise is excellent by itself before bed. Or inhale through right nostril and exhale from left nostril to give yourself clarity, positive mood, and focus more directly. Breathing through both—in the way you're about to learn—helps us garner both sets of benefits. Another way to think about it is that breathing through your left nostril accesses the right side of your brain (your "feeling" brain); breathing in through your right nostril will access the left side of your brain (your "thinking" brain). Consciously moving the breath from side to side through each nostril will help you access your whole brain.

Also, by emphasizing inhaling, the sympathetic part of the autonomic nervous system boosts the heart rate and blood pressure; it boosts alertness and stimulates us, maybe even energizing us.

By emphasizing exhaling, the parasympathetic nervous system slows the heartbeat and relaxes the circulation, nerves, and digestive system. It relaxes us and promotes elimination, both physically and emotionally.

Here are some of the benefits:

- Creates whole brain functioning by balancing the right and left hemispheres. It integrates both sides of the brain, effectively restoring imbalances in the brain.
- Merges the thinking brain and the feeling brain.
- Helps you think more clearly.
- Can help with headaches, migraines, and other stress-related symptoms.
- Improves sleep.
- Cleanses your lungs.
- Regulates the cooling and warming systems of the body.
- Enhances rest and relaxation.

OK, now how do we do it?

- Take a comfortable seat. Allow the spine to stretch tall without becoming overly rigid or tense.
- Do your best to keep the breath relaxed, deep, and full.
- Place your left hand on your lap.
  - If you'd like, you can have the pointer finger and thumb touch each other and the palm up. This is a hand position that subtly encourages focus.
  - The left hand can rest on your thigh throughout the practice.
- Bring the right hand up toward the face. We'll take our pointer finger and middle finger and gently place them on the brow bone at the center of the forehead. The pointer and middle finger can rest here throughout the breath practice.
- Then use the thumb of the right hand to close the right nostril and the ring finger of the right hand to close the left nostril.
- Close the right nostril and gently and fully inhale through the left nostril.

- Then close the left nostril, release the right thumb, and exhale through the right nostril.
- Then inhale through the right nostril.
- Close the right nostril, release the left, and exhale through the left nostril.
- Continue repeating, alternating nostrils after each inhalation.
- This is one round.
- Let's start again and we'll count you through it for a few rounds.
- Start slowly with one or two rounds.
- Close the right nostril and gently and fully inhale through the left nostril for a count of four.
- Then close the left nostril, release the right thumb, and exhale through the right nostril for a count of four.
- Then inhale through the right nostril for a count of four.
- Close the right nostril, release the left, and exhale through the left nostril for a count of four.
- Continue repeating, alternating nostrils after each inhalation. Stick with the four counts, or if you feel it's possible to lengthen the breath and keep it even on both sides, perhaps go to a count of six.
- Sit quietly for a few moments after you have finished.
- Let both hands rest in the lap and breathe in and out through both nostrils.

SQUARE BREATH (SOME PEOPLE CALL IT "TACTICAL BREATHING")

This type of breath work can be done from a few minutes to about 15 minutes.

The breath makes a "square" or a "box" because it is composed of four parts of breath that are all equal in length. We will guide the breath with a four-count inhale, four-count retention (holding the breath in), four-count exhale, and a four-count hold with the breath out. Then we repeat it, counting each piece out silently to ourselves.

Try to keep the face and jaw relaxed when the breath is held. It's easy to tense the face when we concentrate, so just notice if you are and then relax the muscles in the head, face, or neck if you're tensing up. Repeat the four counts on four parts of the breath and continue. Four in. Four hold. Four out. Four hold. (The count of four is not as important as it is that each "piece" or "side" of the breath be equal. If, for instance, you'd like the breath to be longer, then each of the four parts of the breath would be a six count.)

LOVING-KINDNESS MEDITATION FOR COMPASSION

First, we'd like to provide a brief introduction to and background about this type of prayerful meditation. In our typical day-to-day modern life, we might often feel like we are always faced with situations that induce stress, anxiety, frustration, and competing priorities. In these types of intense moments, or as a simple start or end to your day, practicing *loving-kindness*—an ancient form of prayerful meditation—can be really useful to help to "take the edge off." In a best-case scenario, and as you continue with the practice, this meditation may even make it easier to respond to difficult people or situations with empathy and openness, rather than anger and frustration.

The practice is one that aims to cultivate *compassion, appreciative/sympathetic joy*, and *equanimity*. Loving-kindness is similar to benevolence, or the deliverance of goodwill upon others—whether or not they deserve it. This type of practice was developed over 2,500 years ago within the Buddhist tradition, but loving-kindness is practiced worldwide, by a variety of religious and nonreligious people from many traditions.

One of our favorite parts of this meditation is the flexibility it affords and the control we have over the practice. On days that we practice, we feel immense clarity, focus, benevolence, agreeableness, and compassion. You can carry those results with you into the day.

Research suggests that we are not alone.

In 2008, a study from Stanford reported that even an abbreviated loving-kindness induction led to deeper feelings of social connectedness and warmth toward strangers.[1] That same year, colleagues at UNC demonstrated that loving-kindness practice increased adults' social support, purpose in life, mindfulness, and life satisfaction.[2] Post these seminal investigations, numerous other empirical studies have identified additional benefits of cultivating loving-kindness:

- Reduction of repetitive thoughts and decreased symptoms of depression and post-traumatic stress disorder.[3]
- Improvement in back pain, anger levels, and psychological health among sufferers of chronic back pain.[4]
- Improved cognitive processing.[5]

Loving-kindness is not simply a Buddhist tradition. For instance, closely related to it are the Hebrew virtue of *chesed*, the Hindu/Jain value of *ahimsa* ("nonviolence") of which we may be more familiar through our yoga practices, and the Greek concepts of *agape* ("unconditional love") and *theoria* ("loving contemplation"). You don't need to identify yourself as Buddhist, religious, or spiritual to practice and reap the benefits of loving-kindness meditation. All you need is an open mind.

So how exactly does this work?

Here is the basic script we will use for each step of the meditation:

May ___ be happy.
May ___ be healthy.
May ___ be peaceful.
May ___ be loved.

In this progressive meditation, each "blank" represents a particular person. We will guide you through a few rounds.

Please find a comfortable seat or posture lying down if you know you will be able to stay awake, alert, and relaxed. After taking a few deep breaths, there is no need to control your breath. Move your focus from your breath to your heart. You may find it helpful to place one or both of your hands over your heart.

First, deliver self-compassion upon yourself. As you do this, say to yourself with sincerity and clarity, "May I be happy, may I be healthy, may I be peaceful, may I be loved." Allow your breath to freely flow as you repeat these phrases. Allow your breathing to assume a natural pace here. It may be difficult to say these words to yourself or feel these feelings; do your best to acknowledge what you're feeling though. Be kind to yourself in this very process. Repeat "may I be happy, may I be healthy, may I be peaceful, may I be loved." With each breath, let these words and love reach out to every cell in your body: "May I be happy, may I be healthy, may I be peaceful, may I be loved." Be in this loving moment.

Now call to your mind someone you care about. It could be a close friend, a family member, a partner, someone you love very much. Someone for whom you have positive regard. Say their name to yourself. Feel their presence. It may be helpful to visualize this person sitting in front of you. Direct loving-kindness toward this person. "May you be happy, may you be healthy, may you be peaceful, may you be loved." As you say these words, feel the joy in your heart. Feel it as it radiates throughout your body. Visualize it radiating through your body, as well as reaching out toward this person. "May you be happy, may you be healthy, may you be peaceful, may you be loved." With each wish, imagine this person receiving your love, peace, and joy. "May you be happy, may you be healthy, may you be peaceful, may you be loved." Be in this loving moment.

Continue to watch the breath breathe in and out.

Now it potentially gets a little trickier: Think about someone with whom it is challenging or difficult to work, live, or exist. Someone with whom you are experiencing conflict, where there is unhealthy communication. Say their name. Feel their presence. It may be helpful to visualize this person sitting in front of you. Notice if your breath or body changes. Do your best to keep the breath smooth. Then direct loving-kindness toward this person. "May you be happy, may you be healthy, may you be peaceful, may you be loved." Again, this can be difficult, so make sure to be patient. To forgive, to understand, to accept may be difficult. Continue to let these feelings wash over you. Do not be harsh with yourself. Do your best to continue to say, "May you be happy, may you be healthy, may you be peaceful, may you be loved." With each wish, imagine this person receiving your love, peace, and joy. "May you be happy, may you be healthy, may you be peaceful, may you be loved." Be in this loving moment.

Now, bring someone to mind with whom you interact frequently, but do not know very well. It could be perhaps a neighbor or a coworker you don't know well, a waiter or waitress, or a grocer or postal worker. Pick one and visualize that person. Direct loving-kindness toward them. With them in your mind's eye or present in your heart, say to them, "May you be happy, may you be healthy, may you be peaceful, may you be loved." As you repeat these words, feel the joy in your heart. Feel it as it radiates from your heart to every cell of your body. Visualize it radiating out of your body and touching this person. Breathe in and breathe out. "May you be happy, may you be healthy, may you be peaceful, may you be loved." With each wish, imagine this person receiving your love, peace, and joy. "May you be happy, may you be healthy, may you be peaceful, may you be loved." Be in this loving moment.

Now, broaden the scope. For instance, teachers may think about the students and faculty on their campus, or you may consider people in your neighborhood or country; members of your identity groups, such as veterans as a whole or another identity group with which you identify; or even the entire animal kingdom. The basic idea is to extend compassion and goodwill to groups we may or may not know or even like. With that group in mind and in your heart, repeat, "May you be happy, may you be healthy, may you be peaceful, may you be loved." With each wish, imagine this group receiving your love, peace, and joy. "May you be happy, may you be healthy, may you be peaceful, may you be loved." Be in this loving moment.

To conclude, visualize love, kindness, well-being, and peace. Let these radiate from you and your heart toward yourself, toward the person who is close to you, toward the person you have difficulty with, toward the person you don't know but who touches your life, and toward a broader group with which you identify. Wish them all well. Repeat, "May you be happy, may you be healthy, may you be peaceful, may you be loved." Now return to this current space and time. Bring with you the feelings of kindness, peace, love, well-being, and happiness. Carry it with you and share it with others.

When you are ready, open your eyes and stretch out your body.

Congratulations for trying this loving-kindness meditation. Even if this was your first time, know that this, too, is a practice. Try it once, but you will reap the most benefits if you make this a regular practice. You can do it anywhere—in your office, when waiting for a doctor's appointment, or while riding public transportation.

If possible, meditate somewhere quiet and peaceful, free of interruption.

There are many versions of loving-kindness meditation that vary in length, scope, and format. Although a script was provided, you may modify in any way that best suits you. Your task will be to find a method that speaks to you.

NOTES

1. As we have discussed in detail, social connectedness is vital to vibrant human health and positive measurable health outcomes. This specific type of meditation has been well studied and proven to increase feelings of social connectedness. We have taught this specific script to hundreds of veterans in programmatic, formal, and informal settings; every time, we are pleasantly surprised by how well it is received and by the immediate positive impacts noticed by the participants. Hutcherson, C. A., Seppala, E. M., & Gross, J. J. (2008). Loving-kindness meditation increases social connectedness. *Emotion,* 8(5), 720–724.

2. Small changes can make big differences in mental outlook. This meditation has been shown to improve feelings of positivity and connectedness over time and through regular practice. Fredrickson, B. L., Cohn, M. A., Coffey, K. A., Pek, J., & Finkel, S. M. (2008). Open hearts build lives: Positive emotions, induced through loving-kindness meditation, build consequential personal resources. *Journal of Personality and Social Psychology,* 95(5), 1045–1062.

3. Meditation improves feelings of depression or emotional reactivity in study participants. Specifically, this sort of outreach-focused meditation seems to improve symptoms of PTSD. Kearney, D. J., Malte, C. A., McManus, C., Felleman, B., & Simpson, T. L. (2013). Loving-kindness meditation for posttraumatic stress disorder: A pilot study. *Journal of Traumatic Stress,* 26(4), 426–434.

4. This specific form of meditation, like many other types, has been proven to reduce self-reported feelings of pain in participants. Carson, J. W., Keefe, F. J., Lynch, T. R., Carson, K. M., Goli, V., Fras, A. M., & Thorp, S. R. (2005). Loving-kindness meditation for chronic low back pain: Results from a pilot trial. *Journal of Holistic Nursing,* 23(3), 287–304.

5. As chapter 6 highlighted, regulating the nervous system expands working memory capacity. This area of the brain helps with focus and upper-level thinking. In this way, meditation can make a person mentally sharper. Hirshberg, M. J., Goldberg, S. B., Schaefer, S. M., Flook, L., Findley, D., & Davidson, R. J. (2018). Divergent effects of brief contemplative practices in response to an acute stressor: A randomized controlled trial of brief breath awareness, loving-kindness, gratitude or an attention control practice. *PLoS ONE, 13*(12), e0207765.

References

Acosta, J., Adamson, D., Farmer, C., Farris, C., & Feeney, K. C. (2014). *Improving programs that address psychological health and traumatic brain injury: The RAND toolkit.* Santa Monica, CA: RAND Corporation.

Ahmed, S. (2010). *The promise of happiness.* Durham, NC: Duke University Press.

Ajzen, I. (1991). The theory of planned behavior. *Organizational Behavior and Human Decision Processes, 50,* 179–211.

Anderson, J. G., & Taylor, A. G. (2011). Effects of healing touch in clinical practice: A systematic review of randomized clinical trials. *Journal of Holistic Nursing, 29*(3), 221–228.

Andrews-Hanna, J., Smallwood, J., & Spreng, R. (2014). The default network and self-generated thought: Component processes, dynamic control, and clinical relevance. *Annals of the New York Academy of Sciences, 1316,* 29–52.

Barnes, V. A., Monto, A., Williams, J. J., & Rigg, J. L. (2016). Impact of transcendental meditation on psychotropic medication use among active duty military service members with anxiety and PTSD. *Military Medicine, 181*(1), 56–63.

Barrett, B. (2003). Alternative, complementary, and conventional medicine: Is integration upon us? *The Journal of Alternative & Complementary Medicine, 9*(3), 417–427.

Bearman, D., & Shafarman, S. (1999). The Feldenkrais Method in the treatment of chronic pain: A study of efficacy and cost effectiveness. *American Journal of Pain Management, 9,* 22–27.

Becker, I. (2008). Uses of yoga in psychiatry and medicine. In P. R. Muskin (Ed.), *Complementary and alternative medicine and psychiatry* (pp. 107–146). Washington, D.C.: American Psychiatric Press, Inc.

Bensimon, M., Amir, D., & Wolf, Y. (2008). Drumming through trauma: Music therapy with post-traumatic soldiers. *The Arts in Psychotherapy, 35*(1), 34–48.

Bittman, B. B., Berk, L. S., Felten, D. L., Westengard, J., Simonton, C., Pappas, J., & Ninehouser, M. (2001). Composite effects of group drumming music therapy on modulation of neuroendocrine-immune parameters in normal subjects. *Alternative Therapies, 7*(1), 38–47.

Blake, R. L., & Bishop, S. R. (1994). The Bonny Method of Guided Imagery and Music (GIM) in the treatment of post-traumatic stress disorder (PTSD) with adults in the psychiatric setting. *Music Therapy Perspectives, 12*(2), 125–129.

Bormann, J. E., Thorp, S. R., Wetherell, J. L., Golshan, S., & Lang, A. J. (2013). Meditation-based mantram intervention for veterans with posttraumatic stress disorder: A randomized trial. *Psychological Trauma: Theory, Research, Practice, and Policy, 5*(3), 259.

Bossarte, R. M. (Ed.). (2013). *Veterans suicide: A public health imperative* (1st ed.) Washington, D.C.: American Public Health Association.

Bowman, J. (2015). "Wounded warriors": Royal Danish Ballet dancers train repatriated wounded soldiers in Pilates. *Arts & Health, 7*(2), 161–171.

Brenner, L. A., & Barnes, S. M. (2012). Facilitating treatment engagement during high-risk transition periods: A potential suicide prevention strategy. *American Journal of Public Health, 102*, S12–S14.

Burt, J. (1995). Distant thunder: Drumming with Vietnam veterans. *Music Therapy Perspectives, 13*, 110–112.

Cantin, A., & Marshall-Lucette, S. (2011). Examining the literature on the efficacy of equine assisted therapy for people with mental health and behavioural disorders. *Mental Health and Learning Disabilities Research and Practice, 8*(1), 51–61.

Centers for Disease Control and Prevention. (2017). Accessed December 15, 2019, Available at http://www.cdc.gov

Chalmers, J. A., Quintana, D. S., Abbott, M. J., & Kemp, A. H. (2014). Anxiety disorders are associated with reduced heart rate variability: A meta-analysis. *Frontiers in Psychiatry, 5*, 80.

Chapman, J. B., Lehman, C. L., Elliott, J., & Clark, J. D. (2006). Sleep quality and the role of sleep medications for veterans with chronic pain. *Pain Medicine, 7*(2), 105–114.

Chi, I., Jordan-Marsh, M, Guo, M., Xie, B., & Bai, Z. (2013). Tai chi and reduction of depressive symptoms for older adults: A meta-analysis of randomized trials. *Geriatrics & Gerontology International, 13*(1), 3–12.

Church, D. (2013). Clinical EFT as an evidence-based practice for the treatment of psychological and physiological conditions. *Psychology, 4*, 645–654.

Church, D., Hawk, C., Brooks, A. J., Toukolehto, O., Wren, M., Dinter, I., & Stein, P. (2013). Psychological trauma symptom improvement in veterans using emotional freedom techniques: A randomized controlled trial. *The Journal of Nervous and Mental Disease, 201*(2), 153–160.

Clark, M. E. (2004). Post-deployment pain: A need for rapid detection and intervention. *Pain Medicine, 5*(4), 333–334.

Collins, D. A., Shamblen, S. R., Atwood, K. A., Rychener, D. L., Scarbrough, W. H., Abadi, M. H., & Simmons, L. A. (2015). Evaluation of a health coaching course for providers and staff in Veterans Health Affairs medical facilities. *Journal of Primary Care & Community Health, 6*(4), 250–255.

Cooke, B., & Ernst, E. (2000). Aromatherapy: A systematic review. *British Journal of General Practice, 50*(455), 493–496.

Coughlin, S. S. (Ed.). (2012). *Posttraumatic stress disorder and chronic health conditions* (1st ed.). Washington, D.C.: American Public Health Association.

Cumella, E. J., & Simpson, S. (2014). Efficacy of equine therapy: Mounting evidence. *Transactions on Psychology, 1*(1), 13–21.

Currier, J. M., Holland, J. M., & Allen, D. (2012). Attachment and mental health symptoms among U.S. Afghanistan and Iraq veterans seeking health care services. *Journal of Traumatic Stress, 25*(6), 633–640.

Davidson, P. R., & Parker, C. H. (2001). Eye movement desensitization and reprocessing (EMDR): A meta-analysis. *Journal of Consulting and Clinical Psychology, 69*(2), 305–316.

Denneson, L. M., Corson, K., & Dobscha, S. K. (2011). Complementary and alternative medicine use among veterans with chronic noncancer pain. *Journal of Rehabilitation Research and Development, 48*(9), 119–1128.

Department of Defense, Defense Centers of Excellence. (2017, February 20). Holistic therapies help manage stress at home. Accessed February 20, 2017, Available at http://www.dcoe.mil/blog/11-10-20/Holistic_Therapies_Help_Manage_Stress_at_Home.aspx

Department of Veterans Affairs. (2014). *Pain management opioid safety.* Informational brochure.

Department of Veterans Affairs. (2016a). *20161109_CIH for Pain Management at VA_Final V2.docx.* Office of Patient Centered Care and Cultural Transformation. Unpublished memo. Office of Patient Centered Care and Cultural Transformation.

Department of Veterans Affairs. (2016b). *Whole health: OPCC&CT national perspective.* Unpublished presentation. Office of Patient Centered Care and Cultural Transformation.

Department of Veterans Affairs. (2017a). *VA celebrates Global Peer Support Recognition Day.* Accessed March 9, 2017, Available at http://www.blogs.va.gov/VAntage/23497/va-celebrates-global-peer-support-recognition-day/

Department of Veterans Affairs. (2017b). *VA Patient Centered Care.* Accessed February 23, 2017, Available at https://www.va.gov/PATIENTCENTEREDCARE/about.asp

Diamond, D. M., Campbell, A. M., Park, C. R., Halonen, J., & Zoladz, P. R. (2007). The temporal dynamics model of emotional memory processing: A synthesis on the neurobiological basis of stress-induced amnesia, flashbulb and traumatic memories, and the Yerkes-Dodson law. *Neural Plasticity, 2007,* 1–33.

Dobscha, S. K., Corson, K., Flores, J. A., Tansill, E. C., & Gerrity, M. S. (2008). Veterans Affairs primary care clinicians' attitudes toward chronic pain and correlates of opioid prescribing rates. *Pain Medicine, 9*(5), 564–571.

Drescher, K. D., Foy, D. W, Kelly, C., Leshner, A, Schutz, K., & Litz, B. (2011). An exploration of the viability and usefulness of the construct of moral injury in war veterans, *Traumatology, 17* (1), 8–13.

Duhart, O. (2012). PTSD and women warriors: Causes, controls and a congressional cure. *Cardozo Journal of Law & Gender, 18,* 327–331.

Egoscue, P., & Gittines, R. (2014). *Pain free: A revolutionary method for stopping chronic pain.* New York, NY: Bantam.

Elnitsky, C. A., Andresen, E. M., Clark, M. E., McGarity, S., Hall, C. G., & Kerns, R. D. (2013). Access to the US department of Veterans Affairs health system: Self-reported barriers to care among returnees of Operations Enduring Freedom and Iraqi Freedom. *BMC Health Services Research, 13*(1), 1–20.

Emerson, D., Hopper, E., & Levine, P. A. (2011). *Overcoming trauma through yoga: Reclaiming your body.* Berkeley, CA: North Atlantic Books.

Fletcher, D., & Sarkar, M. (2013). Psychological resilience: A review and critique of definitions, concepts, and theory. *European Psychologist, 18*(1), 12–23.

Foa, E. B., Hembree, E. A., & Rothbaum, B. O. (2007). *Prolonged exposure therapy for PTSD: Emotional processing of traumatic experiences, therapist guide.* New York, NY: Oxford University Press.

Foran, H. M., Adler, A. B., McGurk, D., & Bliese, P. D. (2012). Soldiers' perceptions of resilience training and post-deployment adjustment: Validation of a measure of resilience training content and training process. *Psychological Services, 9*(4), 390–403.

Forman, E. M., Herbert, J. D., Moitra, E., Yeomans, P. D., & Geller, P. A. (2007). A randomized controlled effectiveness trial of acceptance and commitment therapy and cognitive therapy for anxiety and depression. *Behavior Modification, 31*(6), 772–799.

Friedman, J. (2015). Risk factors for suicide among Army personnel. *Journal of the American Medical Association. 11*, 1154–1155.

Furlan, A. D., Yazdi, F., Tsertsvadze, A., Gross, A., Van Tulder, M., Santaguida, L, & Skidmore, B. (2011). A systematic review and meta-analysis of efficacy, cost-effectiveness, and safety of selected complementary and alternative medicine for neck and low-back pain. *Evidence-Based Complementary and Alternative Medicine, 2012*, 1–66.

Goertz, C., Marriott, B. P., Finch, M. D., Bray, R. M., Williams, T. V., Hourani, L. L., . . . Jonas, W. B. (2013). Military report more complementary and alternative medicine use than civilians. *The Journal of Alternative and Complementary Medicine, 19*(6), 509–517.

Granath, J., Ingvarsson, S., von Thiele, U., & Lundberg, U. (2006). Stress management: A randomized study of cognitive behavioral therapy and yoga. *Cognitive Behavior Therapy, 35*(1), 3–10.

Gray, M. J., Schorr, Y., Nash, W., Lebowitz, L., Amidon, A., Lansing, A., . . . Litz, B. T. (2012). Adaptive disclosure: An open trial of a novel exposure-based intervention for service members with combat-related psychological stress injuries. *Behavior Therapy, 43*, 407–415.

Greden, J. F., Valenstein, M., Spinner, J., Blow, A., Gorman, L. A., Dalack, G. W., & Kees, M. (2010). Buddy-to-buddy, a citizen soldier peer support program to counteract stigma, PTSD, depression, and suicide. *Annals of the New York Academy of Sciences, 1208*, 90–97.

Gutierrez, P. M., Brenner, L. A., Rings, J. A., Devore, M. D., Kelly, P. J., Staves, P. J., & Kaplan, M. S. (2013). A qualitative description of female veterans' deployment-related experiences and potential suicide risk factors. *Journal of Clinical Psychology, 69*(9), 923–935.

Hayes, S. C., Masuda, A., Bissett, R., Luoma, J., & Guerrero, L. F. (2004). DBT, FAP and ACT: How empirically oriented are the new behavior therapy technologies? *Behavior Therapy, 35*, 35–54.

Hayes, S. C., Wilson, K. G., Gifford, E. V., Bissett, R., Piasecki, M., Batten, S. V., . . . Gregg, J. (2004) A preliminary trial of twelve step facilitation and acceptance and commitment therapy with polysubstance-abusing methadone maintained opiate addicts. *Behavior Therapy, 35*, 667–688.

Heffner, K. L., Crean, H. F., & Kemp, J. E. (2016). Meditation programs for veterans with posttraumatic stress disorder: Aggregate findings from a multi-site evaluation. *Psychological Trauma: Theory, Research, Practice, and Policy, 8*(3), 365–374.

Held, P., & Owens, G. P. (2013). Stigmas and attitudes toward seeking mental health treatment in a sample of veterans and active duty service members. *Traumatology, 19*(2), 136–145.

Hempel, S., Taylor, S. L., Marshall, N. J., Miake-Lye, I. M., Beroes, J. M., Shanman, R., & Shekelle, P. G. (2014). *Evidence Map of Mindfulness.* VA-ESP Project #05-226.

Hempel, S., Taylor, S. L., Solloway, M., Miake-Lye, I. M., Beroes, J. M., Shanman, R., & Shekelle, P. G. (2013). *Evidence Map of Acupuncture.* VA ESP Project #05-226.

Hendricks, K., Turner, L., & Hunt, S. (2014). Integrating yoga into stress-reduction interventions: Application of the health belief model. *Arkansas Journal of Health Promotion, 49*, 55–60.

Henriques, G., Keffer, S., Abrahamson, C., & Horst, S. J. (2011). Exploring the effectiveness of a computer-based heart rate variability biofeedback program in reducing anxiety in college students. *Applied Psychophysiology and Biofeedback, 36*(2), 101–112.

Herbert, M. S., Afari, N., Liu, L., Heppner, P., Rutledge, T., Williams, K., . . . Bondi, M. (2017). Telehealth versus in-person acceptance and commitment therapy for chronic pain: A randomized noninferiority trial. *The Journal of Pain, 18*(2), 200–211.

Hiraoka, R., Cook, A. J., Bivona, J. M., Meyer, E. C., & Morissette, S. B. (2016). Acceptance and commitment therapy in the treatment of depression related military sexual trauma in a woman veteran: A case study. *Clinical Case Studies, 15*(1), 1–14.

Hofmann, S. G., & Smits, J. A. J. (2008). Cognitive behavioral therapy for adult anxiety disorders: A meta-analysis of randomized placebo controlled trials. *Journal of Clinical Psychiatry, 69*(4), 621–632.

Hoge, C. W. (2010). *Once a warrior, always a warrior* (1st ed.). Guilford, CT: Lyons Press.

Hoge, C. W., & Castro, C. A. (2012). Preventing suicides in U.S. service members and veterans. *Journal of American Medical Association, 308*(7), 671–672.

Hoge, C. W., McGurk, D., Thomas, J. L., Cox, A. L., Engel, C. C., & Castro, C. A. (2008). Mild traumatic brain injury in U.S. soldiers returning from Iraq. *New England Journal of Medicine, 358*(5), 453–463.

Ilgen, M. A., McCarthy, J. F., Ignacio, R. V., Bohnert, A. B., Valenstein, M., Blow, F. C., & Katz, I. R. (2012). Psychopathology, Iraq and Afghanistan service, and suicide among Veterans Health Administration patients. *Journal of Consulting and Clinical Psychology, 80*(3), 323–330.

Institute of Medicine (IOM). (2009). *Integrative medicine and the health of the public: A summary of the February 2009 summit.* Washington, D.C.: National Academies Press.

Institute of Medicine (IOM). (2011). *Relieving pain in America: A blueprint for transforming prevention, care, education, and research.* Washington, D.C.: National Academies Press.

International Association of Yoga Therapists. (2017, February 21). Certification Eligibility. Accessed February 15, 2020, Available at http://www.iayt.org /?page=CertifHome

Jain, S, McMahon, G. F., Hansen, P., Kozub, M. P., Porter, V., King, R., & Guarneri, E. M. (2012). Healing Touch with Guided Imagery for PTSD in returning active duty military: A randomized controlled trial. *Military Medicine, 177*(9), 1015.

Jha, A. P., & Kiyonaga, A. (2010). Working-memory-triggered dynamic adjustments in cognitive control. *Journal of Experimental Psychology: Learning, Memory, and Cognition, 36*(4), 1036–1042.

Jha, A. P., Stanley, E. A., & Baime, M. J. (2010). What does mindfulness training strengthen? Working memory capacity as a functional marker of training success. In Bear, R. (Ed.), *Assessing mindfulness and acceptance processes in clients: Illuminating the theory and practice of change,* 207–221. Oakland, CA: New Harbinger.

Jha, A. P., Stanley, E. A., Kiyonaga, A., Wong, L., & Gelfand, L. (2010). Examining the protective effects of mindfulness training on working memory capacity and affective experience. *Emotion, 10*(1), 54–64.

Johnson, D. C., Thom, N. J., Stanley, E. A., Haase, L., Simmons, A. N., Shih, P. A. B., . . . Paulus, M. P. (2014). Modifying resilience mechanisms in at-risk individuals: A controlled study of mindfulness training in Marines preparing for deployment. *American Journal of Psychiatry, 171*(8), 844–853.

Jouper, J., & Johansson, M. (2012). Qigong and mindfulness-based mood recovery: Exercise experiences from a single case. *Journal of Bodywork and Movement Therapies, 17*(1), 69–76.

Kehle-Forbes, S. M., Drapkin, M. L., Foa, E. B., Koffel, E., Lynch, K. G., Polusny, M. A., . . . Oslin, D. W. (2016). Study design, interventions, and baseline characteristics for the substance use and trauma intervention for veterans (STRIVE) trial. *Contemporary Clinical Trials, 50,* 45–53.

Kehle-Forbes, S. M., Meis, L. A., Spoont, M. R., & Polusny, M. A. (2015). Treatment initiation and dropout from prolonged exposure and cognitive processing therapy in a VA outpatient clinic. *Psychological Trauma: Theory, Research, Practice, and Policy, 8*(1), 107–114.

Kobau, R., Seligman, M. P., Peterson, C., Diener, E., Zack, M. M., Chapman, D., & Thompson, W. (2011). Mental health promotion in public health: Perspectives and strategies from positive psychology. *American Journal of Public Health, 101*(8), e1–e9.

Koo, K. H., & Maguen, S. (2014). Military sexual trauma and mental health diagnoses in female veterans returning from Afghanistan and Iraq: Barriers and facilitators to Veterans Affairs care. *Hastings Women's Law Journal, 25*(1), 27–38.

Langmuir, J. I., Kirsh, S. G., & Classen, C. C. (2012). A pilot study of body-oriented group psychotherapy: Adapting sensorimotor psychotherapy for the group treatment of trauma. *Psychological Trauma: Theory, Research, Practice, and Policy, 4*(2), 214.

Lee, L. K., Lee, D., & Woo, J. (2009). Tai chi and health-related quality of life in nursing home residents. *Journal of Nursing Scholarship, 41*(1), 35–43.

Levine, P. (2010). *In an unspoken voice: How the body releases trauma and restores goodness.* Berkeley, CA: North Atlantic Books.

Libby, D. J., Pilver, C. E., & Desai, R. (2012). Complementary and alternative medicine in VA specialized PTSD treatment programs. *Psychiatric Services, 63*(11), 1134–1136.

Lim, E. C. W., Poh, R. L. C., Low, A. Y., & Wong, W. P. (2011). Effects of Pilates-based exercises on pain and disability in individuals with persistent nonspecific low back pain: A systematic review with meta-analysis. *Journal of Orthopaedic & Sports Physical Therapy, 41*(2), 70–80.

Linehan, M. M., Dimeff, L. A., Reynolds, S. K., Comtois, K. A., Welch, S. S., Heagerty, P., & Kivlahan, D. R. (2002). Dialectical behavior therapy versus comprehensive validation therapy plus 12-step for the treatment of opioid dependent women meeting criteria for borderline personality disorder. *Drug and Alcohol Dependence, 67*, 13–26.

Little, P., Lewith, G., Webley, F., Evans, M., Beattie, A., Middleton, K., & Yardley, L. (2008). Randomised controlled trial of Alexander technique lessons, exercise, and massage (ATEAM) for chronic and recurrent back pain. *British Medical Journal, 337*, a884.

Longhofer, J., & Floersch, J. (1993). African drumming and psychiatric rehabilitation. *Psychosocial Rehabilitation Journal, 16*, 3–9.

Malmin, M. M. (2013). Warrior culture, spirituality, and prayer. *Journal of Religion and Health, 52*(3), 740–758.

Meeks, D. W., & Jeste, D. V. (2009). Complementary and alternative medicine in geriatric psychiatry. In B. J. Sadock, V. A. Sadock, & P. Ruiz (Eds.), *Kaplan and Sadock's Comprehensive Textbook of Psychiatry* (pp. 3959–3972). Philadelphia: Lippincott Williams & Wilkins.

Miake-Lye, I. M., Lee, J. F., Luger, T., Taylor, S., Shanman, R., Beroes, J. M., & Shekelle, P. G. (2016). *Massage for Pain: An Evidence Map.* VA ESP Project #05-226.

Nash, William P. (2010). *Moral Injury and Moral Repair: Overview of Constructs and Early Data.* 13th Annual Force Health Protection Conference, Phoenix, AZ, 8/12/10.

Niemtzow, R. C., Belard, J. L., & Nogier, R. (2015). Battlefield acupuncture in the US military: A pain-reduction model for NATO. *Medical Acupuncture, 27*(5), 344–348.

Ogden, P., & Fisher, J. (2015). *Sensorimotor psychotherapy: Interventions for trauma and attachment*. New York, NY: WW Norton & Company.

Ohayan, M. M., & Schatzberg, A. F. (2003). Using chronic pain to predict depressive morbidity in the general population. *American Journal of Psychiatry, 60*(1), 39–47.

Öhman, A., Åström, L., & Malmgren-Olsson, E. B. (2011). Feldenkrais® therapy as group treatment for chronic pain–a qualitative evaluation. *Journal of Bodywork and Movement Therapies, 15*(2), 153–161.

Park, C. L., Finkelstein-Fox, L., Barnes, D. M., Mazure, C. M., & Hoff, R. (2016). CAM use in recently-returned OEF/OIF/OND US veterans: Demographic and psychosocial predictors. *Complementary Therapies in Medicine, 28*, 50–56.

Payne, P., Levine, P. A., & Crane-Godreau, M. A. (2015). Somatic experiencing: Using interoception and proprioception as core elements of trauma therapy. *Frontiers in Psychology, 6*, 93.

Pence, P., Katz, L., Huffman, C., & Cojucar, G. (2014). Delivering integrative restoration-yoga *nidra* meditation (iRest®) to women with sexual trauma at a veteran's medical center: A pilot study. *International Journal of Yoga Therapy, 24*(1), 53–62.

Pereira, L. M., Obara, K., Dias, J. M., Menacho, M. O., Guariglia, D. A., Schiavoni, D., . . . Cardoso, J. R. (2012). Comparing the Pilates method with no exercise or lumbar stabilization for pain and functionality in patients with chronic low back pain: Systematic review and meta-analysis. *Clinical Rehabilitation, 26*(1), 10–20.

Porges, S. W. (2011). *The polyvagal theory: Neurophysiological foundations of emotions, attachment, communication, and self-regulation (Norton Series on Interpersonal Neurobiology)*. New York, NY: W.W. Norton & Company.

Price, C. J., McBride, B., Hyerle, L., & Kivlahan, D. R. (2007). Mindful awareness in body-oriented therapy for female veterans with post-traumatic stress disorder taking prescription analgesics for chronic pain: A feasibility study. *Alternative Therapies in Health and Medicine, 13*(6), 32.

Raingruber, B., & Robinson, C. (2007). The effectiveness of tai chi, yoga, meditation, and reiki healing sessions in promoting health and enhancing problem solving abilities of registered nurses. *Issues in Mental Health Nursing, 28*(10), 1141–1155.

Rankin, L. (2013). *Mind over medicine: Scientific proof you can heal yourself*. Los Angeles, CA: Hay House, Inc.

Rausch, S. M., Gramling, S. E., & Auerbach, S. M. (2006). Effects of a single session of large-group meditation and progressive muscle relaxation training on stress reduction, reactivity, and recovery. *International Journal of Stress Management, 13*(3), 273.

Rubak, S., Sandbaek, A., Lauritzen, T., & Christensen, B. (2005). Motivational interviewing: A systematic review and meta-analysis. *British Journal of General Practice, 55*(513), 305–312.

Saenger, M., Duva, I., & Abraham, C. (2014). "Nurses, Docs, and Drugs" interprofessional facilitation to implement opioid risk mitigation within the patient-centered medical home. *American Journal of Medical Quality, 29*(3), 1–15.

Seal, K. H., Metzler, T. J., Gima, K. S., Bertenthal, D., Maguen, S., & Marmar, C. R. (2009). Trends and risk factors for mental health diagnoses among Iraq and Afghanistan veterans using Department of Veterans Affairs health care, 2002–2008. *American Journal of Public Health, 99*(9), 1651–1658.

Seaward, B. (2004). *Managing stress: Principles and strategies for health and well-being.* Sudbury, MA: Jones & Bartlett.

Seppälä, E. M., Nitschke, J. B., Tudorascu, D. L., Hayes, A., Goldstein, M. R., Nguyen, D. T., & Davidson, R. J. (2014). Breathing based meditation decreases posttraumatic stress disorder symptoms in US Military veterans: A randomized controlled longitudinal study. *Journal of Traumatic Stress, 27*(4), 397–405.

Sherman, K. J., Dixon, M. W., Thompson, D., & Cherkin, D. C. (2006). Development of a taxonomy to describe massage treatments for musculoskeletal pain. *BMC Complementary and Alternative Medicine, 6*(1), 24.

Shiraev, E. B., & Levy, D. A. (2010). *Cross-cultural psychology: Critical thinking and contemporary applications* (4th ed.). Boston, MA: Pearson.

Shulkin, D. J. (2016). Beyond the VA crisis: Becoming a high-performance network. *New England Journal of Medicine, 374*(11), 1003–1005.

Siegel, D. J., & Solomon, M. (Eds.). (2003). *Healing trauma: Attachment, mind, body and brain.* New York, NY: WW Norton & Company.

Slotoroff, C. (1994). Drumming technique for assertiveness and anger management in the short-term psychiatric setting for adult and adolescent survivors of trauma. *Music Therapy Perspectives, 12*, 111–116.

Snyderman, R. (2013). *Reductionism approach.* Duke University Medical Center, Unpublished PowerPoint presentation.

Snyderman, R. (2014). Personalized medicine 2014: Has health care been transformed? *Personalized Medicine, 11*(4), 365–368.

Snyderman, R., & Yoediono, Z. (2006). Prospective care: A personalized, preventative approach to medicine. *Pharmacogenomics, 7*(1), 5–9.

Solloway, M. R., Taylor, S. L., Shekelle, P. G., Miake-Lye, I. M., Beroes, J. M., Shanman, R. M., & Hempel, S. (2016). An evidence map of the effect of Tai Chi on health outcomes. *Systematic Reviews, 5*(1), 126.

Solomon, E. P., & Heide, K. M. (2005). The biology of trauma: Implications for treatment. *Journal of Interpersonal Violence, 20*(1), 51–60.

Spelman, J. F., Hunt, S. C., Seal, K. H., & Burgo-Black, A. L. (2012). Post deployment care for returning combat veterans. *Journal of General Internal Medicine, 27*(9), 1200–1209.

Squier Kraft, H. (2007). *Rule number two: Lessons learned in a combat hospital.* New York, NY: Back Bay Books.

Stanley, E. A., Schaldach, J. M., Kiyonaga, A., & Jha, A. P. (2011). Mindfulness-based mind fitness training: A case study of a high-stress predeployment military cohort. *Cognitive and Behavioral Practice, 18*(4), 566–576.

Stickgold, R. (2002). EMDR: A putative neurobiological mechanism of action. *Journal of Clinical Psychology, 58*(1), 61–75.

Strauss, J. L., Lang, A. J., & Schnurr, P. P. (2017, March 9). PTSD: National Center for PTSD. http://www.ptsd.va.gov/professional/treatment/overview/complementary_alternative_for_ptsd.asp

Tanielan, T., & Jaycox, L. H. (2008). *Invisible wounds of war: Psychological and cognitive injuries, their consequences, and services to assist recovery*. Washington, D.C.: RAND Corporation.

Taylor, P. (2011). *War and Sacrifice in the Post 9/11 Era: The Military-Civilian Gap*. Pew Research Center Social and Demographic Trends, Washington, D.C.

Taylor, S., Bolton, R., Huynh, A., Dvorin, K., Elwy, R., & Bokhour, B. (2019). *Facilitators, challenges and strategies to adopting and implementing Complementary and Integrative Health therapies*. Center for Evaluating Patient-Centered Care in VA. Accessed July 6, 2020, Available at https://www.liebertpub.com/doi/abs/10.1089/acm.2018.0445

Tedeschi, R. G., & Calhoun, L. G. (2004). Posttraumatic growth: Conceptual foundations and empirical evidence. *Psychological Inquiry, 15*(1), 1–18.

Teng, E., Hiatt, E., Mcclair, V., Kunik, M., Stanley, M., & Frueh, B. (2013). Efficacy of posttraumatic stress disorder treatment for comorbid panic disorder: A critical review and future directions for treatment research. *Clinical Psychology: Science and Practice, 20*(3), 268–284.

Thomas, K. H. (2016). Warrior culture. *O Dark Thirty, 4*(2), 47–61.

Thomas, K. H., & Albright, D. L. (Eds.). (2018). *Bulletproofing the psyche: Preventing mental health problems in our military and veterans*. Santa Barbara, CA: ABC-CLIO/Praeger.

Thomas, K. H., Albright, D., Shields, M., Kaufman, E., Michaud, C., Plummer Taylor, S., & Hamner, K. (2016). Predictors of depression diagnoses and symptoms in United States female veterans: Results from a national survey and implications for programming. *Journal of Military and Veterans' Health, 24*(3), 6–17.

Thomas, K. H., & Plummer Taylor, S. (2015). Bulletproofing the psyche: Mindfulness interventions in the training environment to improve resilience in the military and veteran communities. *Advances in Social Work, 16*(2), 312–322.

Thomas, K. H., Plummer Taylor, S., Hamner, K., Glazer, J., & Kaufman, E. (2015). Multi-site programming offered to promote resilience in military veterans: A process evaluation of the Just Roll With it Bootcamps. *Californian Journal of Health Promotion, 13*(2), 15–24.

Thomas, K. H., Turner, L. W., & Kaufman, E., Paschal, A., Knowlden, A. P., Birch, D. A., & Leeper, J. (2015). Predictors of depression diagnoses and symptoms in veterans: Results from a national survey. *Military Behavioral Health, 3*(4), 255–265.

van der Kolk, B. A. (2014). *The body keeps score: Brain, mind, and body in the healing of trauma*. New York, NY: Penguin.

van der Kolk, B. A., & McFarlane, A. C. (Eds.). (2012). *Traumatic stress: The effects of overwhelming experience on mind, body, and society*. New York, NY: Guilford Press.

VanderVaart, S., Gijsen, V. M., de Wildt, S. N., & Koren, G. (2009). A systematic review of the therapeutic effects of Reiki. *The Journal of Alternative and Complementary Medicine, 15*(11), 1157–1169.

Vasterling, J. J., Proctor, S. P., Amoroso, P., Kane, R., Heeren, T., & White, R. F. (2006). Neuropsychological outcomes of army personnel following deployment to the Iraq war. *Journal of the American Medical Association, 296*(5), 519–529.

Walach, H., Güthlin, C., & König, M. (2003). Efficacy of massage therapy in chronic pain: A pragmatic randomized trial. *The Journal of Alternative & Complementary Medicine, 9*(6), 837–846.

Wardell, D. W., Rintala, D., & Tan, G. (2008). Study descriptions of healing touch with veterans experiencing chronic neuropathic pain from spinal cord injury. *Explore: The Journal of Science and Healing, 4*(3), 187–195.

Wilcox, S. L., Finney, K., & Cedarbaum, J. A. (2013). Prevalence of mental health problems among military populations. In B. A. Moore & J. E. Barnett (Eds.), (2013). *Military psychologists' desk reference* (pp. 187–196). New York, NY: Oxford University Press.

Winkelman, M. (2003). Complementary therapy for addiction: Drumming out drugs. *American Journal of Public Health, 93*(4), 647–651.

Wood, D. (2016). *What have we done: Moral injury and our longest wars.* New York, NY: Little, Brown, and Company.

About the Authors and Contributors

KATE HENDRICKS THOMAS, PhD, E-RYT200, is a behavioral health researcher focused on mental health promotion for servicemembers and military veterans. A Master Certified Health Education Specialist (MCHES) and yoga teacher, her interest in veterans' reintegration is informed by her own experiences as a Marine Corps Officer. She is a lecturer in George Mason University's Department of Global and Community Health and is the author of over forty scientific papers, fifty academic conference presentations, and several books on military wellness. Her social commentary and editorials have been featured in *The Washington Post*, *The Hill*, *Task & Purpose*, and Vox Media. Learn more at www.DocKate.com.

SARAH PLUMMER TAYLOR, MSW, E-RYT500, is an established leader in the field of resilience-building, holistic health coaching, and yoga for veterans. Sarah is a former Marine Corps Intelligence Officer who was deployed to Iraq twice and now travels to North America, Central America, and Europe speaking, consulting, offering mindfulness-based programs, and teaching leadership principles. Her work has been featured on Capitol Hill and in news and entertainment outlets such as the *Katie Couric Show*, *NBC Nightly News with Brian Williams*, NPR, MSNBC, and others. Connect with her at www.SemperSarah.com.

JOHN S. HUANG, PhD, is a staff psychologist at the Tibor Rubin VA Medical Center in Long Beach, CA, and also has a private practice. His areas of clinical specialization include diversity issues, meditation/relaxation, depression, and trauma. His interests include Buddhism, Christianity, Hinduism, and Native American spiritualities. He leads a drum circle and teaches tai chi as part of his interest in complementary and alternative medicine. Connect with him at www.drjohnhuang.com.

JUSTIN T. MCDANIEL, PhD, is an Assistant Professor of Public Health in the School of Human Sciences at Southern Illinois University. His primary research interest is the intersection of place of residence, behavioral health, and military service status. He has published over fifty articles in peer-reviewed journals and presented at over thrity conferences, both within the United States and internationally.

PATRICK MCGUIGAN, MS, is the military and veteran legislative assistant for U.S. senator John Boozman (Arkansas). Prior to joining Senator Boozman's team, Pat worked as a professional staff member for the U.S. Senate's Committee for Veterans Affairs, responsible for the committee's oversight on mental health and suicide prevention programs. Before entering public service, Pat served in the Active Duty U.S. Army for thirteen years as a Field Artillery officer. During this time, he served in combat and operational assignments to Iraq; Afghanistan; the 25th Infantry Division, Schofield Barracks, Hawaii; and the 101st Airborne Division, Ft. Campbell, KY.

PAM PENCE, MBA, C-IAYT, E-RYT500, is a yoga therapist focused on delivering the benefits of yoga and meditation to military veterans. She has worked extensively with women healing from military sexual trauma through the Veterans Administration. A Certified iRest Yoga Nidra Meditation Teacher and certified yoga therapist, her affinity for working with veterans stems from her life as a Navy dependent. She teaches yoga *nidra* as part of a yoga therapist certification program at *Be The Change* and is the researcher and author of an article on the impact of yoga *nidra* on the symptoms of military sexual trauma. Contact her at www.MeetYourselfYoga Therapy.com.

Index

Acceptance and Commitment Therapy (ACT), 118, 120, 126

Acupuncture treatments, 56, 116, 128, 132

Agency: as a choice, 21, 23, 50; healing modalities, encouraging experimentation with, 116, 123; health and well-being, agency promoting, 16, 18; individual agency, 54, 117; PTSD diagnosis as sapping feelings of agency, 37; resiliency theory, putting emphasis on agency, 101, 103; yoga as aiding in the cultivation of, 48

Alienation, 9, 33, 68, 77–78

Alternative therapies, 115, 121

Aromatherapy, 130, 133

Battle fatigue, 28, 117

Biofeedback, 84 n.5, 116, 130, 137

Brain: biofeedback, measuring brain waves via, 130; bulletproofing the brain concept, 10, 50, 108, 115; cortisol as interfering with function of, 43, 61; DHEA stress hormone, effect on, 30, 44; emotional regulation and, 31; frontal cortex function and working memory, 41; nervous system regulation, effect on, 35 n.4, 60, 141–142, 148 n.5; prefrontal cortex, prayer causing changes to, 83, 92; rational brain, traumatic memory not found in, 124; resting the brain, 59 n.1, 78, 112–113; re-wiring the brain to ease trauma, 49, 119; stress injuries, effect on, 37; threats, brain activity reacting to, 29; traumatic brain injury, 38

Breathwork: alternate nostril breathing, 141–143; conscious breathing, daily practice of, 56; controlled breath practices, 127; morning breathwork as recommended, 57; as a self-care practice, 54; as a spiritual practice, 81; square breath, tactical breathing through, 50–51, 143–144; working memory, breathwork helping to increase, 59; yoga, as a key component of, 49

Broken veteran narrative, 13, 28, 37, 121–122

Brown, Brené, 83, 85 n.6, 87, 88, 90 n.2

Canadian Forces study on psychological resilience, 102

Chaplaincy as a mental health resource, 82, 84 n.4, 128

Chiropractic care, 56, 131, 132

Civilian world, readjusting to. *See* Transition to civilian life

varying names for, 28; stressors, bodily responses to, 29; veteran community, stress injury rates among, 116; ways to prevent, 115
Suicide: *American Journal of Public Health* study on, 33–34; CIH availability for active duty service members, 135–137; as a public health crisis, 17; resiliency theory, combating suicide rates with, 102, 107–108; separation from service as greatest predictor of, 32, 33, 117; veteran suicide rates, 10, 13, 14, 50
Sympathetic nervous system, 31, 112

Tai Chi, 116, 129, 133
Team Rubicon, 78, 107
Team RWB, 62, 107
Tend and befriend response, 30
Tension, role in mental well-being, 86–87
Therapy animals, 130
Transcendence, rank in Maslow's hierarchy of needs, 83, 91, 114
Transition to civilian life: civilian world, readjusting to, 35, 71 n.2, 98, 107, 109; depression among recently discharged vets, 110, 117; disconnect from civilians, 66, 67–68, 106, 122–123; loss of military community, grieving over, 33–34; modalities popular with the newly transitioning, 132; psychological reintegration, success with, 102–103; resiliency theory, applying during, 98–101; social support of faith communities, 82; stress of transition period, 35 n.6, 109, 137; transition

education, enhancement of, 105; treatment avoidance, changing attitude of, 65–66, 103; warrior culture, as contributing to difficulties with, 14
Tribe, finding or building, 68, 77–78, 113

Veterans Integrated Service Networks (VISNs), 134
Volunteer work, benefits of, 78, 81, 83–84
Vulnerability, cultivating, 75

Warrior culture: assets/strength, favoring over susceptibility/recovery, 99; healing protocols, designing for, 125; peer leadership, importance of, 106; resilience training protocol, 109; resiliency theory, applying to, 101; silent suffering, viewing as a virtue, 8, 14; treatment-stigma issues, 116, 122; whole health model, fitting into, 133
Warrior Wellness Alliance, 107
Werner, Emmy, 99
Wolf, Stuart, 69
Woo, Jean, 129
Working memory capacity, 31, 41, 44, 110 n.4, 136, 148 n.5
Wounded Warrior Project, 107

Yoediono, Ziggy, 117
Yoga: breathwork, practicing in tandem, 48–49, 53–54; chronic pain, treating with, 45–46, 51–52; as a daily practice, 57; effectiveness of, 48, 55; yoga interventions, 45, 125, 128